Post Weight-Loss Surgery Diet

Gastric Bypass Cookbook, Gastric Sleeve Cookbook (Quick And Easy, Before & After, Roux-en-Y, Coping Companion)

Richard P. Russel

Post Weight-Loss Surgery Diet: Gastric Bypass Cookbook, Gastric Sleeve Cookbook (Quick And Easy, Before & After, Roux-en-Y, Coping Companion)

This book was self-published with the amazing help of <u>Self-Publishing Made Easy Now!</u> [1] . You can grab a free copy of the checklist that started my journey here: <u>FREE Self-Publishing Checklist</u> [2] .

[1] https://selfpublishingmadeeasynow.com/xpjv

[2] https://selfpublishingmadeeasynow.com/free_checklist

Table of Contents

Book 1 - Gastric Bypass Cookbook

Quick And Easy Meals After Weight Loss Surgery (Gastric Sleeve, Obesity Related Diseases, Long Term Plan)

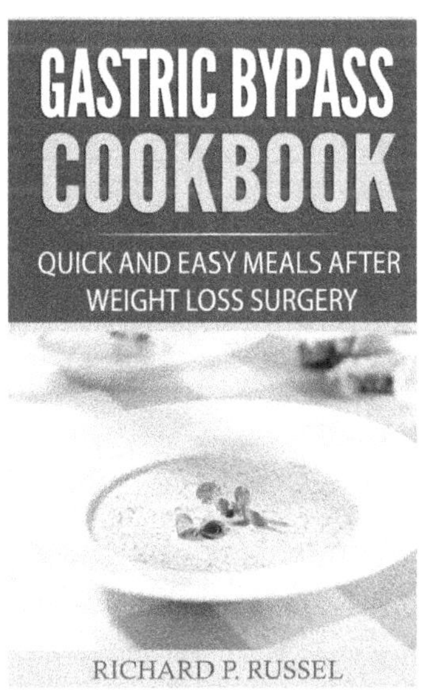

1 - Introduction

Gastric Sleeve Surgery

Gastric sleeve surgery is a non-reversible surgical operation designed to decrease the size of your stomach and help you lose weight. It is an important step you can take to achieve successful weight loss, especially if you are obese or severely overweight and have not lost that weight successfully even after following a diet plan, working out, or taking medicine.

Smaller is Better

Having a smaller stomach means you will be satisfied with what you are eating more quickly. Now that you have a smaller tummy, it also means you have to change certain things related to the way you eat, such as consuming foods in portion sizes that are smaller than what you have been used to so that you can easily reach your weight loss goals.

Making the Cut

In carrying out the gastric sleeve operation, the surgeon either goes for an open operation where he makes a big incision in your abdomen or uses the laparoscopic approach in which he makes a number of small incisions with the aid of a camera and small instruments.

Either way, you will end up having a large part of your stomach (more than half) removed, and with a banana-sized tube (thin vertical sleeve) left. To help your newly reduced stomach after the operation, surgical staples are put in place.

An Instant Fix It Is Not

Your doctor will generally consider you as a candidate for gastric sleeve surgery when your BMI (body mass index) hits the 40 or 40-plus mark. This operation is also an option your doctor might resort to if you suffer from a disabling or life-threatening condition on top of having a BMI of 35 or higher.

All of these sound hopeful, but you need to realize that gastric sleeve surgery is a weight loss tool, not an operation that will instantly fix your excess weight woes. Even with the help of going through a gastric sleeve surgical operation, you will still have to follow a healthy diet plan and engage in regular physical activity. Otherwise, you will just gain back all of that lost weight.

Pretty Effective

As shown in research studies, gastric sleeve surgery can help you people shed off more than ½ of their excess pounds.

Individuals who are more realistic in their weight loss goals and expectations also have a higher success in terms of the amount of weight lost, especially if they make sure to keep on eating their recommended diet plan, being physically active, and keeping their appointments with their health care/medical team.

The Ever After

What to eat will most likely be your greatest concern after going through your gastric sleeve surgery. Expect your doctor to provide you a detailed list of what you can and what you cannot eat after the operation. For the first post-surgery month, during which your body is on healing mode, you smaller stomach will only be able to hold soft foods as well as liquids in small amounts.

You need to keep hydrating your body during this period, which you easily accomplish by sipping water all through the day. You will probably realize that your bowel movements become irregular after the operation – although this is a common outcome of gastric sleeve surgery, it is important that you avoid bowel movement straining and constipation.

You will find that you can gradually include solid foods into your after-surgery diet plan. Take extra care to really chew your food, and always stop eating anything the moment you feel full. This does take some getting used to, especially when you feel satisfied after consuming food in fewer quantities than what you have been accustomed to.

If you forget to chew your food well and keep on eating after you feel full, you may experience nausea and discomfort, which can sometimes be accompanied by vomiting. If you consume plenty of fruit juices, sodas, or other high-calorie beverages, you may be able to reach your weight loss goals.

And if you keep on overeating, your reduced stomach may get stretched, which will cancel out the benefits brought on by your gastric sleeve operation.

Your doctor may encourage you to seek the advice of a dietitian who can help you create and follow a healthy diet plan that allows your body to lose weight while still getting adequate protein as well as vitamins and minerals. It is important to stick to your new diet and make sure to keep on taking your recommended supplemental vitamins and minerals.

2 - Obesity-Related Diseases

Gastric sleeve surgery will not only help you lose weight, it will also help you avoid suffering from various health conditions related to obesity, such as type 2 diabetes, gallbladder disease, gout, stroke and heart disease, cancer, osteoarthritis, and sleep apnea. A person is considered obese when he or she weighs at least twenty percent more than his or her normal weight.

Diabetes (type 2)

Most individuals suffering from diabetes (type 2) are usually also suffering from overweight or obesity. Reduce your risk of developing this condition by shedding off those excess pounds, following a balanced diet plan, engaging in regular physical exercise, and making sure to get enough sleep.

If you do suffer from diabetes (type 2), make sure to lose weight as well as get more physical exercise so that you can get your blood sugar levels stabilized. When your body is more active, you will find that you have less need for taking your medication to treat diabetes.

Gallbladder disease

Being overweight increases your chances of developing gallstones and gallbladder disease. Keep in mind though, that losing weight may actually cause your body to form gallstones. To get around this irony, make sure to lose weight following a target rate of no more than one pound per week.

Gout

Your joints are the ones affected by gout, and this disease is a result of your blood having high levels of uric acid. All that excess uric acid in your bloodstream can crystallize and get lodged in your joints.

In the same ironic vein as the gallstones, your gout condition may actually flare up when you experience sudden weight loss. To get around this problem, make sure to get your doctor's advice on how to lose weight.

Stroke and heart disease

Carrying excess weight in your body can increase your risk of having high cholesterol levels and suffering from high blood pressure, both of which can also may it more likely for you to have a stroke or get heart disease.

Fortunately, you can lose weight to decrease your risk of suffering from stroke or heart disease. Even if you just lose five to ten percent of your weight, it is enough so that your risk of developing heart disease will be decreased.

Cancer

Aside from being linked by a number of studies to pancreatic cancer, ovarian cancer, and cancer of the gallbladder, obesity is also linked to colon cancer as well as cancers of the kidney, esophagus, breast (post-menopause), and endometrium or uterine lining.

Osteoarthritis

When you have osteoarthritis, your back, hip, or knee is affected. Osteoarthritis results from your excess weight placing added pressure on the said joints, which cause their cartilage (joint-cushioning tissue) to get worn away. By losing extra weight, you help ease the stress on your joints in the lower back, hips, and knees, as well as improve your osteoarthritis symptoms.

Sleep apnea

Being overweight can lead to a breathing condition called sleep apnea, in which the individual affected snores heavily in his or her sleep and then suddenly stops breathing for a brief moment. This can cause you to feel sleepy during the day as well as increase your risk of having stroke and heart disease. If you have sleep apnea, losing weight can help you improve your condition.

3 - Long-Term Habits

Undergoing a gastric bypass surgery helps you control your calorie intake, adopt proper eating habits, and achieve your weight loss goals. The following tips should enable you to eat and thrive after surviving your surgery.

Take enough liquids (six to eight cups daily is recommended) to hydrate your body properly. Try the following:

- Drink 1 cup of fluid over an hour.

- Don't drink anything within thirty minutes to one hour of a meal.

- Make sure to slowly sip your allowed liquids.

- Never use a straw when drinking your liquids.

Consume adequate amounts of protein.

Supplement your gastric bypass diet with the necessary vitamins and minerals once your doctor allows you to. Make sure to take calcium, iron, zinc, and B12 supplements.

Steer clear of all forms of high-calorie foods and drinks.

Eat your food really slowly and thoroughly.

Once you feel full, stop eating. You will know you are full when:

- You feel pressure in the middle just beneath the rib cage.

- You feel nauseous.

- You feel a shoulder or upper chest pain.

Begin each meal with protein. Your pouch will eventually expand, and then you will only need to consume three meals plus one to two protein-rich snacks every day.

Avoid the following foods, which you may find difficult to handle, after the surgery:

- Peas, dried beans, cabbage, celery, corn, and other fibrous vegetables; raw vegetables; and mushrooms

- Coconut, dried fruits, grapefruit and orange membranes, and all fruit peels/skins

- Pork chops and other fatty meat cuts, as well as fried meats, fish, and poultry

- Hamburger, steak, and other meat substitutes

- Starches including granola, non-toasted bread (white/whole grain), cereals (whole grain), bran and bran cereals, popcorn, and noodle/vegetable soups

- Sweets like desserts, sweetened fruit juice, sweetened beverages, jam/jelly, and candy

- Nuts and seeds

- Pickles

- Spiced foods and other highly seasoned foods

- Carbonated drinks

Depending on your tolerance and making sure to advance gradually, follow the 5-Phase Weight Loss Surgery Diet in the next chapter.

4 - 5-Phase Weight Loss Surgery Diet

1st Phase – Clear Liquid Diet

1. Until your surgeon approves it, you should not consume any food or drink any beverage after your gastric sleeve operation.

2. As soon as your surgeon does approve, expect to drink water, broth (clear), apple juice (unsweetened), tea (decaffeinated), and other non-red fluids. You can drink only one ounce or thirty milliliters of liquid per hour. If you find that you can handle drinking one ounce per hour, you can then drink up to two ounces or sixty milliliters of liquid per hour the next day.

3. Never use a straw, which will cause you to drink your liquids too quickly. "Slowly" should be your keyword when it comes to drinking liquids.

4. Know that you are not expected to drink every liquid brought to you down to the last drop. As soon as your stomach feels full, stop drinking.

5. You may experience nausea, vomiting, or both during

your first post-gastric sleeve surgery days. This is not uncommon and is no cause for alarm – just remember to drink slowly. Immediately contact a nurse if the vomiting or nauseous feeling does not go away.

2nd Phase – Full Liquid Diet

1. The day you are discharged from the hospital is the day you can get started on your full liquid diet phase.

2. Unless your surgeon, as well as a dietitian, advises otherwise, you need to be in the 2nd phase (full liquid) diet for a period of one to two weeks.

3. Keep nausea and vomiting at bay by making sure to slowly drink your liquids. See to it that you sip two ounces or one-fourth cup of liquid in more than thirty minutes. But you should force yourself to drink up everything – stop as soon as you feel full.

4. Between your high-protein drinks, make sure to take in a minimum of six to eight cups of drinking water or beverages that are low in calories. Steer clear of citrus, caffeinated, and carbonated drinks.

5. As instructed, do not forget to take your supplemental calcium, multivitamins, and minerals.

6. Monitor your intake of all high-protein drinks, including their kinds and amounts. Make sure to reach your target of sixty grams of protein per day.

3rd Phase – Puree Diet

1. Once you are done with your one- to two-weeks' worth of full liquid diet, you can gradually include thicker consistency-foods to your gastric sleeve diet. Make sure to blend or puree all your foods for the following two weeks to the consistency of baby foods.

2. You have the option of incorporating your full liquid diet foods into your puree (3rd phase) diet.

3. Remember to always chew your foods carefully, which will help in preventing feelings of nausea or blockage. Check first if you can handle eating one to two tablespoons of pureed foods at a time. See to it that your every meal is composed of just two to four tablespoons or one-eighth to one-fourth cup of food.

4. Never forget to consume protein first in each of your meals. Make sure to get at least sixty grams of protein into your body on a daily basis.

5. Hydrate your body by making sure to drink six to eight cups of water as well as low-calorie drinks before and after meals. You can have a portion of your overall fluid intake consist of one-percent or fat-free milk.

6. Keep monitoring your protein intake on a daily basis, taking note of of their kinds and amounts.

4th Phase – Soft Diet

1. After having done the two-week long puree diet, there is no longer a need for you to keep blending your food. Slowly introduce soft-consistency foods to your diet, making sure you can easily cut them with a fork.

2. Keep in mind that the soft (4th phase) diet lasts for two weeks, during which you can try eating new food one at a time.

3. You will find controlling your portions much easier if

you eat off smaller plates. It also helps to use baby spoons and bay forks. Don't forget to stop eating as soon as you feel full.

4. Make sure your body is always hydrated. Between meals, strive to drink six to eight cups of water/low-calorie drinks. But do not drink your liquids with your meals – you can have your liquids half an hour before and half an hour after your meal.

5. Remember to keep taking your prescribed supplements.

6. Keep monitoring your kinds and amounts of protein consumed each day. You should aim to eat at least sixty grams of protein every day.

5th Phase – Regular Diet

1. You should be ready to follow the regular (5th phase) diet after two weeks on your soft (4th phase) diet. You may be able to take up the regular diet one month or two months after surgery, depending on your post-gastric sleeve surgery body's progress.

2. You can keep on slowly introducing new foods during this phase of your diet. You may add vegetables and fruits, but you might be better off avoiding any fruit skins and membranes.

3. Make sure to keep your diet low in fats and free of simple sugars. Remember that your protein consumption should be sixty grams or more daily. To help you lose weight successfully, keep your intake of calories in the range of eight hundred to one thousand two hundred per day (consult your dietitian on the appropriate amount of calories that suits your needs).

4. Remember to keep eating five to six small meals daily. It may be better for you to have three small meals as well as one to two snacks (high-protein) per day as your new stomach expands.

5. Keep taking your prescribed supplements (you will be taking them for life).

6. Always hydrate yourself by drinking six to eight cups of water as well as low-calorie drinks every day.

7. Keep monitoring your daily food consumption as well as activities, taking note of your calorie intake, protein intake, fluid intake, supplements, and physical activity.

8. Keep track of any warning signs your body may be sending. Your new stomach may not be comfortable taking in some food or have yet to get used to portion sizes right. Make sure to watch out for these symptoms and consequently modify your diet:

Feeling full

Prior to your gastric sleeve surgery, it felt normal for you to feel full after eating. Post-surgery, however, you should strive to avoid feeling full before you stop eating. This is an effective way for you to steer clear of any vomiting problems.

Nausea/vomiting

A food you ate may be the reason for your nausea or vomiting, although being dehydrated can also play a part, especially when it occurs quickly and rarely. Make sure to note the food you ate in your food journal for future reference, and always drink sixty-four ounces of fluids on a daily basis.

Bloating/cramping

Certain food may be the culprit for your bloating or cramping. Take note of what you ate and exclude it from your diet; otherwise, cook it using another cooking method.

Chest pain/discomfort

Write down the food you ate as well as its amount in your food journal right away. If your chest pain or discomfort does not subside immediately or if it keeps coming back after every meal, call your doctor as soon as possible.

Abdominal pain/continual vomiting

This warrants an immediate call to your doctor. This could be a signal of surgery complications, so get medical attention right away. It may be nothing, or it may be serious, but it is always better to be safe than sorry when it comes to your health.

5 - Chicken Recipes

Balsamic Rosemary Chicken Roast

Ingredients:

- Rosemary, fresh (1 tablespoon) OR dry (1 teaspoon)

- Rosemary sprigs, fresh (8 pieces)

- Olive oil, extra virgin (1 tablespoon)

- Brown sugar (1 teaspoon)

- Chicken, whole (4 pounds)

- Garlic clove (1 piece)

- Black pepper, freshly ground (1/8 teaspoon)

- Balsamic vinegar (1/2 cup)

Directions:

1. Set the oven at 350 degrees to preheat.

2. Place the garlic and rosemary (both minced) in a medium bowl. Mix well and set aside.

3. Loosely separate the skin of the chicken from its flesh. Rub the flesh with the olive oil before rubbing with the rosemary-garlic mixture as well. Sprinkle on the black pepper and then fill the chicken's cavity with two sprigs of rosemary.

4. Truss the chicken before placing inside a roasting pan. Roast in the preheated oven for about one hour and twenty minutes, making sure to baste the chicken frequently with the juices in the pan. Once the juices run clear and the meat is browned, remove the chicken from the oven and place on a platter. Set aside.

5. Meanwhile, pour the balsamic vinegar as well as brown sugar into a saucepan. Heat on medium and stir the mixture without boiling or until the sugar is completely dissolved.

6. Remove the skin off the chicken after carving it. Pour the vinegar mixture onto the carved chicken pieces, then top with the rest of the rosemary sprigs.

7. Serve right away.

Braised Mushrooms and Chicken

Ingredients:

- Black pepper, freshly ground (1/2 teaspoon)

- Chicken legs, skinless (2 pieces)

- Stock/broth, chicken/vegetable, low sodium (3/4 cup)

- Thyme, fresh, chopped (2 tablespoons)

- Thyme sprigs, fresh (3 pieces)

- Chicken breast halves, bone-in, sliced crosswise (4 pieces)

- Mushrooms, white button, small, brushed clean (1 pound)

- Balsamic vinegar (2 tablespoons)

- Flour, all-purpose (1/4 cup)

- Olive oil, extra virgin (1 ½ tablespoons)

- Chicken thighs, bone-in, skinless (2 pieces)

- Shallots, chopped (1 tablespoon)

- Pearl onions, peeled (1/2 pound)

- Red wine, dry (1/2 cup)

- Salt (1/4 teaspoon)

Directions:

1. Place the flour in a small bowl. Add the pepper (1/4 teaspoon) and mix well.

2. Add the chicken pieces to the seasoned flour, turning to coat them evenly on all sides.

3. Heat a large saucepan (heavy bottomed) on medium-high before adding the oil. Add the coated chicken pieces and cook for two to three minutes on each side or until cooked through and browned. Place on a platter and set aside.

4. Stir shallot into the same saucepan. Cook for one minute or until softened, then stir in the mushrooms.

Cook for an additional three to four minutes or until lightly browned.

5. Add the onions, stir well, and cook for another two to three minutes or until a bit browned.

6. Pour in the wine and stock. Stir and scrape until the pan is deglazed. Add back the chicken pieces and allow to boil before covering and turning the heat down to low. Simmer the mixture for about forty to forty-five minutes or until the veggies and chicken are tenderly cooked.

7. Add in the chopped thyme, salt (1 teaspoon), remaining pepper (1/4 teaspoon), and vinegar. Stir to combine.

8. Arrange the vegetables in warmed individual bowls. Add the chicken pieces (2 pieces per bowl) on top before garnishing with sprigs of thyme.

9. Serve and enjoy.

Cheesy Chicken Wrap

Ingredients:

- Onions, chopped (1/4 cup)

- Tortilla, whole wheat, low carb (1 piece)

- Mushrooms, sliced (1/4 cup)

- Hot chili peppers, pickled, sliced (2 teaspoons)

- Chicken breast, skinless, boneless, w/ fat trimmed out (1/4 pound)

- Green pepper, sliced (1/4 cup)

- Swiss cheese, wedged slice, ¾-ounce (1 piece)

Directions:

1. Pound the chicken breast until about a quarter-inch thick, then slice thinly into strips. Set aside.

2. Heat a large skillet (nonstick) on medium before misting lightly with cooking spray. Once hot, add the onion as well as the chicken strips. Cook for about

five minutes or until the chicken pieces are cooked through and the onions are fragrant and translucent.

3. Stir in the mushrooms and green peppers. Cook for two minutes or until softened, then set aside.

4. Insert the tortilla between two paper towels (dampened with a little water). Heat in the microwave for about twenty seconds, then lay flat on a plate.

5. Spread cheese evenly down the center of the warm tortilla, then top with the chicken strips as well as the mushrooms, onions, peppers, and chili peppers.

6. Fold the tortilla before serving. Enjoy.

Chicken and Cabbage Salad

Ingredients:

- Chicken breasts, boneless, skinless (1 ¼ pounds)

- Lemongrass stalks, w/ 6-inches bottom only, sliced thinly (2 pieces)

- Soy sauce, reduced sodium (1 tablespoon)

- Olive oil, extra virgin (3 tablespoons)

- Peanuts, dry roasted, unsalted, crushed (1 tablespoon)

- Spring onion, sliced into lengthwise halves (1 piece)

- Green onions, sliced thinly (2 pieces)

- Rice vinegar (2 tablespoons)

- Peanut butter (1 tablespoon)

- Cabbage head, green, small (1/2 piece)

- Stock/broth, chicken/vegetable, reduced sodium (2 cups)

- Ginger, fresh, sliced thinly, ½-inch (1 piece)

- Cilantro sprigs, fresh (3 pieces)

- Cilantro, fresh, chopped (3 tablespoons)

- Lime juice, freshly squeezed (2 tablespoons)

- Fish sauce (1 tablespoon)

- Shallot, minced (1 tablespoon)

- Garlic clove (1 piece)

- Spinach (1/2 bunch)

- Carrot, large, peeled, sliced into lengthwise halves, cut diagonally into thin slices (1 piece)

Directions:

1. Fill a large saucepan with the stock as well as ginger, cilantro, lemongrass, and green onion. Stir to combine and heat on high. Allow the mixture to boil before reducing heat to low, then simmer for about five minutes.

2. Stir in the chicken breasts. Return the heat to high to allow the mixture to boil again.

3. Turn heat back to low and let the mixture simmer for about three minutes. Remove from heat, uncover, and let the chicken sit in the stock until slightly cooled.

4. Pour the stock into a large bowl and set aside. Meanwhile, shred the chicken into half-inch-thick and two-inch-long strips. Place in the refrigerator.

5. After straining off the solids from the cooled stock, pour the stock (1½ cups) back into the saucepan. Heat on medium-high and allow the stock to boil for five to six minutes, uncovered, or until reduced to 1/3 its original volume.

6. Fill a blender with the reduced stock. Add in the vinegar, soy sauce, lime juice, fish sauce, garlic, shallot, and peanut butter. Process until well-combined and evenly smooth. Gradually stream in the olive oil as you keep the blender motor running. Set aside the now-thinner dressing.

7. Meanwhile, discard the spinach stems and core the cabbage. Chop the spinach crosswise into quarter-inch strips and place in a large bowl; repeat with the cabbage (add to the same bowl as the spinach).

8. Add the shredded chicken to the spinach-cabbage bowl. Add in the carrot, green onions, and cilantro as well. Gently toss to combine.

9. Top the salad with the prepared dressing (1/2 portion) before dividing among salad plates.

10. Serve garnished with peanuts, alongside the remaining dressing.

Easy Chicken Rollantini

Ingredients:

- Breadcrumbs, whole wheat, Italian seasoned (1/2 cup)

- Ricotta cheese, part skim (6 tablespoons)

- Egg whites, divided (6 tablespoons)

- Marinara sauce (1 cup)

- Chicken breast cutlets, 3-ounces, pounded until thin (8 pieces)

- Parmesan cheese, grated, divided (1/4 cup)

- Spinach, frozen, thawed, squeezed of liquid until dry (5 ounces)

- Mozzarella cheese, part skim, shredded, divided (6 ounces)

- Cooking spray, nonstick

Directions:

1. Set the oven at 450 degrees to preheat.

2. Meanwhile, use cooking spray to grease a glass baking dish (9x13). Set aside.

3. Place chicken cutlets in a large bowl. Add the pepper and salt; rub on the chicken pieces to season well. Set aside.

4. Place the breadcrumbs and Parmesan cheese (2 tablespoons) in a medium bowl. Stir to combine before setting aside.

5. Fill another medium bowl with the egg whites (1/4 cup). Set aside.

6. Place mozzarella cheese (1 ½ ounces) in a large bowl. Add the remaining Parmesan cheese as well as ricotta cheese and remaining egg whites (2 tablespoons).

7. Arrange the seasoned cutlets on a large tray. Add the spinach-cheese mixture (2 tablespoons) on top of each chicken piece, making sure to spread evenly.

8. Roll each chicken cutlet as you loosely keep their seams down, then use a toothpick to secure each cutlet.

9. Place each rolled chicken piece in the egg white mixture, then dredge in the breadcrumbs mixture. Arrange all coated chicken rolls in the prepped baking dish and then lightly coat with cooking spray (non-stick).

10. Place in the oven to bake for twenty-five minutes. Once done, remove from the oven and smother with the marinara sauce. Top with the shredded mozzarella cheese and return to the oven to bake for another three minutes.

11. Once the cheese on top has melted, remove the dish from the oven and sprinkle with Parmesan cheese. Serve immediately.

Healthy Chicken Pizza

Ingredients:

- Pizza crust, thin, 12-inch (1 piece)

- Chicken breast, cooked, sliced into one-inch thickness, w/ visible fat trimmed off (4 ounces)

- Tomato, sliced (1 piece)

- Mozzarella cheese, reduced fat, shredded (1 cup)

- Tomato sauce, w/out added salt (1 cup)

- Green pepper rings (8 pieces)

- Mushrooms, sliced (1 cup)

- Barbecue sauce, homemade (4 tablespoons)

Directions:

1. Set the oven to 400 degrees to preheat.

2. Cover the entire surface of the pizza crust with the sauce, making sure to evenly spread the sauce. After

drizzling the barbecue sauce on top, sprinkle with the shredded mozzarella cheese.

3. Place in the oven to bake for about twelve to fourteen minutes.

4. Once done, remove from the oven and slice into eight portions.

5. Serve and enjoy.

Smokin' Chicken Fajitas

Ingredients:

- Garlic cloves, minced (2 pieces)

- Onion, large, sliced (1 piece)

- Salsa (1/2 cup)

- Cumin, ground (1/2 teaspoon)

- Bell pepper, sweet, red, slivered (1/2 piece)

- Cheese, low fat, shredded (1/2 cup)

- Lime juice, freshly squeezed (1/4 cup)

- Chili powder (1 teaspoon)

- Chicken breasts, skinless, boneless, sliced into quarter-inch strips (3 pounds)

- Bell pepper, green sweet, slivered (1/2 piece)

- Tortillas, whole wheat, 8" (12 pieces)

- Sour cream, fat free (1/2 cup)

Directions:

1. Place chicken strips in a large mixing bowl. Add the slivered bell peppers, minced garlic, ground cumin, chili powder, and lime juice. Toss until well-combined and the chicken strips are evenly coated.

2. Cover the bowl and place in the refrigerator. Allow the chicken to marinate for about fifteen minutes.

3. Heat a large saucepan on medium after spraying generously with nonstick cooking spray. Add the marinated chicken and cook for about three minutes or un-

til cooked through.

4. Add the peppers and onions. Stir and cook for three to five minutes or until soft and fragrant.

5. Spoon equal portions of the prepared chicken mixture onto each tortilla.

6. Top each fajita with two teaspoons each of salsa, sour cream, and shredded cheese before rolling up.

7. Serve and enjoy.

Spinach Stuffed Cajun Chicken

Ingredients:

- Jack cheese, reduced fat, shredded (3 ounces)

- Cajun seasoning (2 tablespoons) – see below

- Chicken breasts, skinless, boneless (1 pound)

- Spinach, frozen, thawed, drained OR fresh cooked (1 cup)

- Bread crumbs, whole wheat (1 tablespoon)

Cajun seasoning:

- Oregano (1/4 teaspoon)

- Onion powder (3/4 teaspoon)

- White pepper (1/4 teaspoon)

- Black pepper (1/4 teaspoon)

- Thyme (1/4 teaspoon)

- Paprika (3/4 tablespoon)

- Garlic powder (3/4 teaspoon)

- Cayenne pepper (1/2 teaspoon)

- Cumin (1/4 teaspoon)

Directions:

1. Set the oven at 350 degrees to preheat. Meanwhile, use tin foil to line a baking sheet; set aside.

2. Pound the chicken on a cutting board until about a quarter of an inch in thickness.

3. Place the spinach in a large bowl. Add the Jack cheese, pepper, and salt, then toss to combine.

4. Place the breadcrumbs in a medium bowl. Add the Cajun seasoning and mix well.

5. Top each chicken breast with the spinach mixture (1/4 cup) before rolling tightly and securing the seams with toothpicks.

6. Brush olive oil onto each stuffed chicken roll, then sprinkle with the prepared breadcrumbs mixture. After making sure each chicken roll is evenly covered, add the rest of the cheese and spinach on top.

7. Arrange the stuffed chicken pieces inside the lined baking sheet and place in the oven to bake for about thirty-five to forty minutes or until the chicken pieces are completely cooked.

8. Remove the baking sheet from the oven, take out the toothpicks, and transfer the stuffed chicken onto a platter.

9. Slice into medallions and serve right away.

10. Enjoy.

Tasty Chicken Lettuce Wraps

Ingredients:

- Water chestnuts, drained, minced (8 ounces)

- Soy sauce, low sodium (2 teaspoons)

- Onion, minced (1 cup)

- Sesame oil, toasted (1 teaspoon)

- Hoisin sauce (2 tablespoons)

- Stevia (2 packets)

- Green onion, whole, chopped (1 piece)

- Bamboo shoots, drained, minced (8 ounces)

- Cooking wine, sherry (3 tablespoons)

- Peanut butter, unsalted (1 tablespoon)

- Hot pepper sauce (2 teaspoons)

- Garlic, minced (1 tablespoon)

- Chicken breast, ground (1/2 pound)

- Salt (1/4 teaspoon)

- Butter lettuce leaves, small (8 pieces)

- Cucumber, small, seeded, sliced into one-inch strips (1 piece)

Directions:

1. Place the bamboo shoots in a large bowl. Add the sherry, peanut butter, hot pepper sauce, hoisin sauce, soy sauce, sugar substitute, and water chestnuts. Stir to combine before setting aside.

2. Heat a large skillet (nonstick) on medium after misting it with cooking spray. Stir in the onion to cook for about four minutes or until softened and fragrant.

3. Stir in the garlic; cook for one minute before turning the heat up to medium-high. Stir in the salt, ginger, and ground chicken. Cook for three to four minutes or until the chicken is cooked through and broken up.

4. Stir in the bamboo shoot mixture and cook for an additional two to three minutes. Add the toasted sesame oil. Give everything a good stir before turning off the heat.

5. Top each lettuce leaf with equal portions of the chicken mixture, then top with cucumber and chopped green onion.

6. Serve right away.

Yummy Chicken Casserole

Ingredients:

- Chicken breast, skinless, cooked, cubed (1 cup)

- Mushrooms, canned (4 ounces)

- Soup, cream of chicken, 98-percent fat free (10 ½ ounces)

- Pepper, freshly cracked (1/4 teaspoon)

- Garlic powder (1/4 teaspoon)

- Onion powder (1/4 teaspoon)

- Pasta, whole wheat, uncooked (1/2 cup) OR cooked (1 cup)

- Mixed vegetables, frozen (2 cups)

- Cheddar cheese, 2-percent milk, reduced fat, shredded (1 cup)

- Water (3/4 cup)

Directions:

1. Set the oven at 350 degrees to preheat.

2. Use cooking spray to coat a casserole dish (9x13).

3. Follow package directions in cooking the vegetables and pasta.

4. Place the chicken in a large mixing bowl. Add the mushrooms, cheese (1/2 cup), water, soup, and milk as well as the cooked vegetables and pasta. Gently toss to combine, making sure the veggies and pasta are evenly coated.

5. Stir in the onion powder, garlic powder, and pepper

before pouring the entire mixture into the prepped casserole dish. Top with the remaining cheese and place in the preheated oven.

6. Bake for about twenty-five to thirty minutes or until the cheese turns bubbly and golden.

7. Serve and enjoy.

6 - Fish Recipes

Alfredo Salmon

Ingredients:

- Salmon fillets, 4-ounces (4 pieces)

- Garlic cloves, minced (4 pieces)

- Salt (1/2 teaspoon)

- Broth, chicken, low sodium, warmed (1 cup)

- Parmesan cheese, grated (1/2 cup)

- Olive oil, extra virgin (1 tablespoon)

- Milk, skim (2 cups)

- Flour, all purpose (3 tablespoons)

- Black pepper, freshly ground (1/4 teaspoon)

Directions:

1. Heat a medium-size saucepan (nonstick) on medium before adding the olive oil.

2. Stir in the garlic and cook for two minutes or until fragrant.

3. Add the flour, stirring continuously until it thickens into a paste.

4. Pour in the warmed chicken broth and whisk well to combine.

5. Stir in the milk along with the pepper and salt.

6. Reduce heat to low and allow the mixture to cook until nicely thickened and smooth.

7. Add the Parmesan cheese; stir into the mixture before serving immediately.

Barbecued Salmon Roast

Ingredients:

- Lemon juice, freshly squeezed (2 tablespoons)

- Lemon rind, grated (2 teaspoons)

- Cinnamon (1/4 teaspoon)

- Brown sugar (2 tablespoons)

- Salt (1/2 teaspoon)

- Pineapple juice (1/4 cup)

- Salmon fillets, 6-ounces (4 pieces)

- Chili powder (4 teaspoons)

- Cumin, ground (3/4 teaspoon)

Directions:

1. Set the oven at 400 degrees to preheat.

2. Fill a large Ziploc bag with the pineapple juice, brown sugar, and salmon fillets. Gently toss inside the bag to combine, then place in the refrigerator to marinate for one hour, turning the bag halfway.

3. Once the salmon fillets are done marinating, take out of the bag (discard the remaining marinade) and transfer onto a plate.

4. Stir the rest of the ingredients together in a large bowl. Once combined, rub over the salmon fillets.

5. Arrange the fillets inside the prepped baking dish. Place in the oven to bake for about twelve to fifteen minutes or until done.

6. Garnish with sliced lemon and serve immediately.

Broiled Roughy Fillets

Ingredients:

- Lemon wedges, medium (8 pieces)

- Dijon mustard (1 tablespoon)

- Pepper, freshly ground (1/4 teaspoon)

- Lemon juice, freshly squeezed (3 tablespoons)

- Olive oil, extra virgin (1 tablespoon)

- Roughy fillets, orange, 4-ounces (4 pieces)

Directions:

1. Tent a broiler pan's rack with tin foil before spraying with nonstick cooking spray. Set aside.

2. Pour olive oil into a medium bowl. Add the mustard, ground pepper, and lemon juice. Stir to combine.

3. Arrange the roughy fillets on the prepped rack. Take ½ of the mustard mixture (set aside the rest for using later) and brush on the fillets.

4. Cook the fillets under the broiler for about five minutes or until the flesh easily flakes.

5. Sprinkle the remaining mustard mixture on the broiled roughy fillets; season with pepper and salt.

6. Garnish with lemon wedges before serving immediately.

7. Enjoy.

Cornmeal Crusted Fish Fillets

Ingredients:

- Olive oil, extra virgin (2 teaspoons)

- Cornmeal, yellow (3 tablespoons)

- Celery seeds, ground (1/4 teaspoon)

- Salt (1 pinch)

- Fish fillets (8 ounces)

- Parsley, chopped (1 ½ tablespoons)

- Black pepper, freshly ground (1/4 teaspoon)

Directions:

1. After cleaning and rinsing the fish fillets, and checking if no bones are left in their flesh, gently pat dry with paper towels. Set aside on a plate.

2. Place the cornmeal in a large bowl. Add the chopped parsley, pepper, celery seed, and salt. Stir to combine.

3. Pour the cornmeal mixture on top of the fish fillets. Make sure all sides of the fish are covered before carefully pressing the cornmeal onto the fillets.

4. Meanwhile, heat a nonstick skillet on medium before adding the olive oil. Once heated through, add the fillets and cook for about two to three minutes on each side or until crisp and brown on the outside and flaky on the inside.

5. Serve and enjoy.

Dill Relished Bass

Ingredients:

- Sea bass fillets, white, 4-ounces (4 pieces)

- Baby capers, pickled, drained (1 teaspoon)

- Dijon mustard (1 teaspoon)

- White onion, chopped (1 ½ tablespoons)

- Dill, fresh, chopped (1 ½ teaspoons)

- Lemon juice, freshly squeezed (1 teaspoon)

- Lemon, sliced into quarters (1 piece)

Directions:

1. Set the oven to 375 degrees to preheat.

2. Meanwhile, fill a medium bowl with the dill, mustard, capers, lemon juice, and onion. Stir to combine.

3. Cut 4 squares of aluminum foil. Fill each square with

one sea bass fillet and moisten with some lemon juice. Top with the dill mixture (1/4 portion per fillet) before wrapping the ends of the foil around the fillet.

4. Bake in the oven for about ten to twelve minutes or until opaque and cooked through.

5. Serve and enjoy.

Easy and Crunchy Tuna Patties

Ingredients:

- Egg whites (4 pieces)

- Onion, minced (1 tablespoon)

- Carrot, grated (1/4 cup)

- Pepper, freshly cracked (1/4 teaspoon)

- Dill (1/4 teaspoon)

- Mustard, dried (1/4 teaspoon)

- Tuna, canned, packed in water (12 ounces)

- Water chestnuts/ red pepper/ capers, chopped (1/4 cup)

- Crackers, wheat, thin, crushed (16 pieces)

Directions:

1. Place the tuna and all the remaining ingredients in a large bowl. Toss to combine.

2. Mold the tuna mixture into 8 equal sized patties.

3. Use cooking spray (nonstick) to coat a skillet (medium size). Heat on medium before adding the tuna patties.

4. Cook for about two to three minutes on each side or until cooked through and golden brown.

5. Serve and enjoy.

Greek Yogurt Salmon Fillets

Ingredients:

- Greek yogurt, plain, nonfat (1 cup)

- Garlic powder (1 teaspoon)

- Seasoning salt (1 ½ teaspoons)

- Salmon fillets, 4-ounces (4 pieces)

- Parmesan cheese, grated (1/2 cup)

- Pepper, freshly cracked (1/2 teaspoon)

Directions:

1. Set the oven to 375 degrees to preheat.

2. Place the cheese in a large bowl. Add the seasonings and Greek yogurt. Stir to combine.

3. Use foil to line a baking sheet, then lightly coat with cooking spray.

4. Dip the salmon fillets in the Greek yogurt mixture, making sure they are evenly coated.

5. Arrange the coated fillets on the prepped baking sheet. Bake in the oven for forty-five minutes or until done.

6. Serve and enjoy.

Lemon-Caper Cod

Ingredients:

- Lemons (2 pieces)

- Tap water, hot (1 cup)

- Flour, all purpose (1 tablespoon)

- Cod fillets, 6-ounces (4 pieces)

- Bouillon granules, chicken flavored, low sodium (1 teaspoon)

- Butter, soft (1 tablespoon)

- Capers, rinsed, drained (4 teaspoons)

Directions:

1. Set the oven at 350 degrees to preheat.

2. Meanwhile, use cooking spray to lightly coat 4 foil squares on the surface. Set a single piece of cod fillet

at the center of each foil square, then drizzle with lemon juice from half a piece of lemon. Slice the remaining half piece of lemon and place on top of the fish pieces.

3. Seal each of the filled foil square before placing in the oven. Bake for about twenty minutes or until the fish pieces are cooked through and opaque.

4. Meanwhile, carefully remove the peel off the other lemon, making sure none of the pith is removed as well. Cut the removed peel into quarter-inch-wide slices and place in a small bowl.

5. Pour hot tap water into another small bowl. Stir in the granulated chicken bouillon; once all the granules are completely dissolved, set aside.

6. Place the flour in a large bowl. Add the butter and stir to combine. Once evenly mixed, pour into a saucepan (heavy bottomed). Heat on medium and stir the flour-butter mixture continuously. Once thickened, stir in the capers and immediately turn off the heat.

7. Pour the thickened flour-butter mixture on top of the

fish. Add the lemon peel slices and serve right away.

Salmon with Mushroom Gravy

Ingredients:

- Sage, fresh, w/ stem discarded, chopped finely (2 tablespoons)

- Milk, skim (1 cup)

- Salmon fillets, 4-ounces (4 pieces)

- Soup, cream of mushroom, unsalted, divided (4 cups)

- Thyme, fresh, w/ stem discarded, chopped finely (2 tablespoons)

- Cornstarch (1/4 cup)

Directions:

1. Pour the cream of mushroom soup into a large saucepan. Heat on medium and stir continuously until heated through. Stir in the thyme and sage, then simmer until the soup is reduced to about ¾ its original volume. Turn off the heat and set aside.

2. Fill a medium bowl with the milk. Stir in the cornstarch. Once well-combined, pour into the simmering mushroom soup and stir well.

3. Allow the mixture to boil before stirring continuously for about three to five minutes or until thickened. Transfer into a gravy boat and set aside.

4. Meanwhile, heat a large saucepan (nonstick). Add a little olive oil and the salmon fillets. Cook for two to three minutes on each side or until cooked through and flaky.

5. Serve the salmon fillets smothered with the mushroom gravy.

Teriyaki Grouper

Ingredients:

- Garlic, minced (1/2 teaspoon)

- Teriyaki sauce, reduced sodium (1 tablespoon)

- Grouper fillets, 4-ounces (2 pieces)

- Italian seasoning (1/4 teaspoon)

- Lemon wedges (2 pieces)

Directions:

1. Fill a medium bowl with the garlic and teriyaki sauce. Whisk well to combine, then brush this mixture on all sides of the grouper fillets.

2. Use cooking spray to lightly coat a baking pan. Add the teriyaki-brushed grouper fillets at the bottom.

3. Cover the pan and place in the refrigerator to marinate for a minimum of fifteen minutes.

4. Meanwhile, turn on the broiler (grill) to preheat before positioning the rack about four inches away from the source of heat.

5. Cook the fish for about five to ten minutes or until the flesh is opaque and slightly firm.

6. Once done, take the fish out of the broiler and immediately sprinkle with the lemon juice from one wedge as well as Italian seasoning.

7. Serve and enjoy.

7 - Shrimp Recipes

Creamy Shrimp Salad

Ingredients:

- Pickle juice (1 tablespoon)

- Eggs, powdered (1 tablespoon)

- Mayonnaise, homemade (1 ½ tablespoons)

- Shrimp, large, shelled, deveined, poached (6 ounces)

Directions:

1. Set the poached shrimp on a platter. Set aside.

2. Fill a blender with the powdered eggs, pickle juice, and homemade mayonnaise. Process until evenly combined and smooth.

3. Pour the creamy dressing over the shrimp.

4. Serve and enjoy.

Cucumber Yogurt Shrimp

Ingredients:

- Lemon juice, freshly squeezed (3 tablespoons)

- Cucumbers, medium, peeled, seeded, diced (2 pieces)

- Dill, chopped finely (1 tablespoon)

- Greek yogurt, plain, fat free (3 cups)

- Garlic, chopped (1 clove)

- Salt (1 tablespoon + a dash)

- Pepper, freshly cracked (a dash)

- Shrimp, large, shelled, deveined, poached (4 ounces)

Directions:

1. After peeling the cucumbers, slice into lengthwise halves. Scrape out the flesh with a spoon before discarding the seeds.

2. Chop the cucumber flesh into cubes, then place in the

colander. Combine with salt (1 tablespoon) and let sit for half an hour.

3. After draining the cucumber pieces, wipe dry with paper towels and place inside the food processor.

4. Pour lemon juice into the food processor. Add in the black pepper, garlic, and dill as well. Process until the mixture is well-blended and smooth, then transfer into a large bowl.

5. Add in the yogurt. Stir to combine. Refrigerate for two to five hours or until all the flavors are blended.

6. Set the poached shrimp on a serving platter.

7. Remove the cucumber yogurt mixture from the refrigerator and pour over the shrimp.

8. Serve and enjoy.

Honey-Glazed Shrimp with Avocado-Strawberry Salad

Ingredients:

- Shrimp, large, shelled, deveined (16 ounces)

- Spring lettuce mix, fresh (6 cups)

- Avocado, sliced into cubes (1 piece)

- Cheese, feta/ Gorgonzola, crumbled (4 ounces)

- Strawberries, hulled, sliced (1 pint)

- Red onion, small, sliced thinly (1/4 piece)

- Almonds, sliced, toasted (1/4 cup)

Glaze:

- Honey (1 tablespoon)

- Liquid smoke (1 teaspoon)

- Olive oil, extra virgin (2 tablespoons)

- Lemon juice, freshly squeezed (1 tablespoon)

- Sea salt (1/4 teaspoon)

Dressing:

- Balsamic vinegar (2 tablespoons)

- Dijon mustard (1 teaspoon)

- Sea salt (1/4 teaspoon)

- Black pepper, freshly ground (1/4 teaspoon)

- Olive oil, extra virgin (1/4 cup)

- Honey (1 tablespoon)

- Garlic powder (1/4 teaspoon)

Directions:

1. Pour the honey in a medium bowl. Add the lemon juice, olive oil, salt, and liquid smoke. Stir to combine; set aside.

2. Set the grill on medium-high to preheat.

3. Meanwhile, rinse the shrimp well. Pat dry with paper towels before brushing with olive oil. Arrange on the preheated grill and cook on each side for about four to five minutes.

4. Once the shrimp pieces are done, transfer onto a plate and brush the tops with the prepared glaze.

5. Arrange equal portions of the spring mix among four individual plates. Add the avocado, strawberries and red onion, then top with the sliced almonds and cheese.

6. Meanwhile, pour the ingredients for the dressing in a medium bowl. Stir to combine before pouring over the salad plates.

7. Top each dressed salad with the glazed shrimp and serve immediately.

8. Enjoy.

Pesto Shrimp

Ingredients:

- Shrimp, large, shelled, deveined, poached (4 ounces)

- Garlic cloves, minced (2 pieces)

- Spinach, frozen, thawed, drained well, chopped (10

ounces)

- Basil, fresh (1/3 cup)

- Olive oil, extra virgin (1 tablespoon)

- Water (1/2 cup)

- Cottage cheese, 1-percent (1/3 cup)

- Parmesan cheese, grated (2 tablespoons)

Directions:

1. Fill the blender with the spinach.

2. Add the garlic, basil, cheeses, olive oil, and water.

3. Process until well-combined and smooth.

4. Arrange the shrimp into a mound on a platter. Drench with the pesto.

5. Serve immediately.

Romaine Shrimp Salad

Ingredients:

- Garlic cloves, minced (2 pieces)

- Baby spinach leaves, fresh, whole (3 cups)

- Kalamata olives (1/3 cup)

- Lemon zest, freshly grated (1/2 teaspoon)

- Tomatoes, medium, sliced thinly into wedges (2 pieces)

- Feta cheese, reduced fat (1/4 cup)

- Shrimp, large, fresh/ frozen, peeled, deveined (1 pound)

- Butter, melted (1 tablespoon)

- Sea salt (1/4 teaspoon)

- Romaine lettuce, torn (3 cups)

- Cucumber, medium, peeled, sliced lengthwise into quarters about ¼-inch thick (1 piece)

- Red onion, chopped (1/4 cup)

Vinaigrette:

- Vinegar, red wine (1 tablespoon)

- Oregano, fresh, chopped (1 tablespoon)

- Agave nectar (1 tablespoon)

- Black pepper, freshly ground (1/4 teaspoon)

- Olive oil, extra virgin (3 tablespoons)

- Lemon juice, freshly squeezed (1 tablespoon)

- Mint, fresh, chopped (1 tablespoon)

- Sea salt (1/2 teaspoon)

Directions:

1. Get the grill ready. Meanwhile, rinse the shrimp before patting dry with several sheets of paper towels.

2. Stir together the butter, garlic, salt, and lemon zest in a large bowl. Add the shrimp and toss with the butter mixture to combine. After seeing to it that the shrimp pieces are evenly coated, cover the bowl and set aside

for about thirty minutes.

3. In another large bowl, toss the spinach and romaine with the olives, tomatoes, red onion, and cucumber. Let sit as you continue working on the shrimp.

4. Thread the butter mixture-coated shrimp onto four skewers (8-inch), making sure they are spaced about ¼-inch apart. Cook on the grill for about six to eight minutes or until opaque. Arrange on a platter and set aside.

5. In a medium bowl, combine the ingredients for the vinaigrette. Process with an immersion blender until evenly mixed and smooth.

6. Top the greens on the platter with feta cheese. Add the grilled shrimp before drizzling with the prepared vinaigrette.

7. Serve and enjoy.

Shrimp and Cranberry Stuffing

Ingredients:

- Celery, chopped (1 cup)

- Tarragon, died (1 teaspoon)

- Water chestnuts, whole (1 cup)

- Bread slices, whole wheat, toasted, sliced into one inch cubes (10 pieces)

- Nutmeg, ground (1/8 teaspoon)

- Shrimp, large, shelled, deveined, poached (8 ounces)

- Chicken broth, low sodium (1 cup)

- Onion, chopped (1/2 cup)

- Parsley, fresh, chopped (1/4 cup)

- Paprika (1/2 teaspoon)

- Cranberries, fresh, chopped (1/2 cup)

- Apple, chopped (1 cup)

Directions:

1. Set the oven at 350 degrees to preheat. Meanwhile,

use cooking spray to lightly coat a baking dish (2-quart).

2. Heat a large skillet (nonstick) on medium after filling it with the chicken broth.

3. Stir in the onion and celery. Allow the mixture to cook for about five minutes or until the veggies are tender. Turn off the heat, add the poached shrimp, and let the mixture sit.

4. Place the bread cubes in a large mixing bowl. Add the water chestnuts, chopped apples, and cranberries as well as tarragon, nutmeg, parsley, and paprika. Toss to combine before stirring in the onion-celery mixture.

5. Transfer the shrimp and cranberry stuffing into the prepped dish. Cover with foil before placing in the oven.

6. Bake for about twenty minutes, then remove the foil cover. Return to the oven and bake for another ten minutes.

7. Serve right away.

Shrimp Enchilada

Ingredients:

- Shrimp, large, shelled, deveined, poached (2 cups)

- Enchilada/ taco sauce, canned, divided (1 cup)

- Mexican cheese, reduced fat, shredded (1/2 cup)

- Scallions, medium, white + green portions, chopped (6 pieces)

- Pinto beans, canned, drained, rinsed (15 ounces)

- Tortillas, medium, low carb, fat free (4 pieces)

Directions:

1. Set the oven at 350 degrees to preheat. Meanwhile, slightly coat a baking dish (9x13) with nonstick cooking spray.

2. Place the turkey in a large bowl. Add the beans, enchilada/taco sauce (1/2 cup), and scallions. Stir to

combine.

3. Add ¼ of the turkey mixture onto each tortilla. Enclose the fillings by folding up the top, bottom, and sides.

4. Arrange the filled tortillas inside the prepped baking dish, making sure to place them with their seam-sides facing down.

5. Top the enchiladas with the remaining enchilada/ taco sauce (1/2 cup) before sprinkling on the cheese.

6. Use aluminum foil to cover the dish before placing in the oven to bake. After twenty minutes or once the cheese is all melted and bubbly, remove from the oven and serve immediately.

Shrimp Rolls

Ingredients:

- Basil pesto, homemade (1/4 cup)

- Bread crumbs, panko (2 tablespoons)

- Olive oil, extra virgin (1 tablespoon)

- Garlic cloves, minced (2 pieces)

- Sea salt (1/4 teaspoon)

- Black pepper, freshly ground (1/4 teaspoon)

- Pecans, chopped finely (1/4 cup)

- Lemon zest, freshly grated (1/2 teaspoon)

- Shrimp, large, shelled, deveined (16 ounces)

- Carrot, shredded (1/4 cup)

Directions:

1. Set the oven at 375 degrees to preheat.

2. Meanwhile, use cooking spray (nonstick) to coat a baking dish (11x7). Set aside.

3. Rinse the shrimp, then pat dry with paper towels. Spread basil pesto (1 tablespoon) onto one side before topping with shredded carrot (1 tablespoon). Loosely roll up each shrimp and secure with a tooth-

pick.

4. Place all loosely rolled up shrimp pieces at the bottom of the prepped dish. Brush olive oil on top.

5. Meanwhile, place the panko breadcrumbs in a large bowl. Add the pecans, garlic, pepper, salt, and lemon zest. Mix well before pressing onto the olive oil-brushed surfaces of the shrimp rolls.

6. Place in the oven to bake for about ten to fifteen minutes or until the shrimp is opaque and the crust is browned.

7. Serve immediately.

Spinach with Lemon-Grilled Shrimp

Ingredients:

- Garlic cloves, minced (2 pieces)

- Black pepper, freshly ground (1/4 teaspoon)

- Baby spinach, packed loosely, washed, dried (5 cups)

- Butter, melted (1 tablespoon)

- Milk, half and half, fat free (1/4 cup)

- Pine nuts, toasted (1/4 cup)

- Shrimp, large, shelled, deveined (1/2 pound)

- Lemon zest, freshly grated (1 tablespoon)

- Lemon juice, freshly squeezed (3 tablespoons)

- Salt (1/2 teaspoon)

- Mascarpone cheese (1/4 cup)

- Nutmeg, freshly grated (1/4 teaspoon)

- Parmesan cheese, shaved (1/4 cup)

Directions:

1. Get the grill ready.

2. Meanwhile, pat the shrimp dry after rinsing well. Place inside a large bowl and toss with salt, pepper, garlic, butter, lemon juice, and lemon zest. Cover and set aside for half an hour.

3. Thread the shrimp pieces onto two skewers (8-inch), making sure to leave a quarter inch of space in between each piece. Arrange the skewered shrimp on the grill to cook for about six to eight minutes or until opaque.

4. Meanwhile, pour the milk into a medium bowl. Add the nutmeg and mascarpone and whisk well until evenly combined. Transfer the mascarpone sauce into a large pot.

5. Heat the pot on low. Stir the mascarpone sauce as you add in the spinach. Once the spinach is wilted, pour in some pasta water (2 tablespoons) and allow the mixture to cook for two more minutes or until the spinach leaves are cooked.

6. After seasoning the spinach mixture with pepper and salt, pour into a serving bowl. Add pine nuts on top, then sprinkle with Parmesan cheese. Finish off by topping everything with the grilled shrimp.

7. Serve and enjoy.

8 - Turkey Recipes

Easy Herbed Turkey

Ingredients:

- Thyme, dried (1 tablespoon)

- Water (1/2 cup)

- Sage, dried (2 teaspoons)

- Parsley, fresh, chopped (2 tablespoons)

- Olive oil, extra virgin (1 tablespoon)

- Turkey, whole, thawed, 15-pounds (1 piece)

Au jus:

- Thyme, dried (1 tablespoon)

- Honey (2 tablespoons)

- Pan drippings, defatted (1 cup)

- Sage, dried (2 teaspoons)

- Parsley, fresh, chopped (2 tablespoons)

- Apple juice (1/2 cup)

Directions:

1. Set the oven at 325 degrees to preheat. Meanwhile, combine the parsley, thyme, and sage in a small bowl; set aside.

2. Discard the turkey's neck and giblets. Use cool water to rinse the turkey thoroughly inside and out, then use paper towels to pat it dry.

3. Gently loosen the neck skin with your fingers before placing the turkey on a roasting pan's rack, making sure to position it breast-side up. Place the herb mixture (1 tablespoon) beneath each breast skin, then rub the turkey's exterior with olive oil and then the rest of the herb mixture.

4. Secure the turkey legs by loosely tying together before placing the turkey in the oven's middle part. Cook for one hour and thirty minutes before tenting with foil. Cook for another two hours or until nicely roasted, with the juices running clear.

5. Once done, take the turkey out of the oven and let sit for twenty minutes.

6. While the turkey juices are settling in the cooling meat, stir half a cup of water into the skillet (heated on medium-high) as you scrape up the remaining browned turkey bits. Pour into a small bowl, leaving one cup of the drippings in the pan. Add the apple juice, honey, sage, parley, and thyme; stir to combine. Reduce heat to medium and simmer the mixture until reduced to half its original volume.

7. Slice the turkey and serve drizzled with the prepared au jus. Enjoy.

Mouthwatering Turkey Turnovers

Ingredients:

- Turkey meat, ground, breast meat part only (1 pound)

- Crescent rolls, reduced fat, refrigerated (24 pieces)

- Onion soup, dry (1 envelope)

- Cheese, 2-percent low fat, shredded (1 cup)

Directions:

1. Set the oven to 350 degrees to preheat. Meanwhile, line a cookie sheet with parchment paper; set aside.

2. Heat a large skillet (nonstick) on medium after misting with cooking spray. Add the meat and dry onion soup. Stir to combine, then cook until the meat is browned and cooked through.

3. Stir in the cheese. Set aside to cool slightly.

4. Separate the rolls before slicing into halves shaped into triangles.

5. Fill each triangle center with the prepared meat mixture, then fold and seal before arranging on the lined cookie sheet.

6. Place in the oven to bake for fifteen minutes.

7. Serve and enjoy.

Slow Cooked Creamy Turkey

Ingredients:

- Soup, cream of mushroom, reduced fat (10 ¾ ounces)

- Chicken stock (1/2 cup)

- Mushrooms, packaged (8 ounces)

- Turkey breast, boneless, skinless (6 pieces)

- Cottage cheese, pureed (1 cup) OR Greek yogurt, plain, nonfat (1 cup)

- Dressing mix, Italian (0.7 ounces)

Directions:

1. Mist cooking spray on a large skillet (nonstick). Heat on medium-high, then add the turkey breasts. Cook on each side for about two to three minutes or until lightly browned.

2. Once the turkey breasts are done, place in the slow cooker (5-quart).

3. Meanwhile, pour the chicken stock and cream of mushroom soup into the skillet, then stir in the

Italian dressing mix and Greek yogurt/cottage cheese. Heat on medium and allow the mixture to cook for two to three minutes as you stir constantly, or until the mixture is well-blended and smooth.

4. Top the slow cooker turkey with the mushrooms, then submerge with the prepared soup mixture. Cover to cook for four hours on low heat.

5. Give the slow cooker turkey mixture a good stir. Serve and enjoy.

Stir-Fried Eggplant and Turkey

Ingredients:

- Mint, fresh, chopped (2 tablespoons)

- Ginger, peeled, chopped (1 tablespoon)

- Bell pepper, red, seeded, julienned (1 piece)

- Soy sauce, low sodium (2 tablespoons)

- Spring onions, white & green parts, chopped coarsely (2 pieces)

- Spring onions, white & green parts, sliced thinly (1 piece)

- Eggplant, small, unpeeled, diced (4 cups)

- Turkey breasts, boneless, skinless, sliced into two-inch-long & half-inch-wide strips (1 pound)

- Basil, fresh, chopped coarsely (1/4 cup)

- Broth/ stock, turkey/ chicken, low sodium (3/4 cup)

- Garlic cloves (2 pieces)

- Olive oil, extra virgin (2 tablespoons)

- Yellow onion, chopped coarsely (1/2 cup)

- Bell pepper, yellow, seeded, julienned (1 piece)

Directions:

1. Fill a blender with the stock (1/4 cup). Add the garlic, ginger, green onions, mint, and basil. Process until just minced, then set aside.

2. Heat a large frying pan (nonstick) on medium-high.

Add olive oil (1 tablespoon), then stir in the yellow onion, bell peppers, and eggplant. Cook for about eight minutes or until the vegetables are nicely sautéed and tender. Place inside a large bowl and keep warm by covering with paper towels.

3. Pour the rest of the olive oil (1 tablespoon) into the pan and heat on medium-high. Stir in the basil mixture; constantly stir for one minute before stirring in the soy sauce and turkey strips as well. Saute for about two minutes or until the meat is opaque and cooked through.

4. Pour in the remaining stock (1/2 cup). Stir and allow to boil before adding back in the eggplant mixture. Stir the entire mixture for about three minutes or until everything is heated through.

5. Pour the stir-fried turkey-eggplant mixture onto a serving dish (warmed). Serve garnished with green onion slices.

6. Enjoy.

Stuffed Turkey Breasts

Ingredients:

- Onion, chopped (1/2 cup)

- Apple, peeled, chopped (1 cup)

- Milk, fat free (1 cup)

- Lemon, sliced into four wedged pieces (1 piece)

- Garlic, minced (1/4 teaspoon)

- Turkey breast halves, large, w/ bones removed, 6-ounces (4 pieces)

- Flour, all purpose (2 tablespoons)

- Raisins, seedless (3 tablespoons)

- Celery, chopped (1/2 cup)

- Bay leaf (1 piece)

- Water chestnuts, chopped (2 tablespoons)

- Olive oil, extra virgin (2 tablespoons)

- Curry powder (1 teaspoon)

Directions:

1. Set the oven at 425 degrees to preheat.

2. Use cooking spray to coat a large baking dish; set aside.

3. Place the raisins in a small bowl. Pour in warm water to cover and allow the raisins to stay submerged until swelling.

4. After misting cooking spray on a large skillet, heat on medium. Add the garlic, onions, bay leaf, and celery; stir and cook for five minutes or until onions are translucent. Discard the bay leaf before stirring in the apples. Let the mixture cook for two more minutes.

5. After draining the raisins, dry by patting with paper towels. Stir into the apple mixture, along with the water chestnuts. Turn off the heat and allow the mixture to cool.

6. Meanwhile, slightly tug at the turkey breast skin to loosen. Insert the apple mixture into the space between the turkey breast and skin.

7. Heat a new skillet on medium. Add the olive oil; once hot, add the stuffed turkey breasts. Cook on each side for about five minutes or until browned and cooked through.

8. Place the browned turkey breasts at the bottom of the prepped baking dish. Cover and place in the oven to bake for about fifteen minutes or until the internal temperature of the meat reaches 165 degrees. Take the dish out of the oven and set aside.

9. Fill a saucepan with the milk. Stir in the flour and curry powder, then heat on medium. Keep stirring for five minutes or until the mixture has thickened, then immediately pour on top of the stuffed turkey pieces.

10. Cover the dish and bake again for about ten minutes before placing the stuffed turkey breasts on individual plates (warmed). Drench the tops with the prepared milk mixture. Add the lemon wedges and serve right away.

Turkey and Beans

Ingredients:

- Basil, dried (2 teaspoons)

- Navy beans, rinsed, drained (16 ounces)

- Black pepper, freshly cracked (1/4 teaspoon)

- Basil leaves, fresh/ dried (a handful)

- Turkey breast halves, skinless, boneless, sliced into lengthwise cuts (2 pieces)

- Salt (1/4 teaspoon)

- Bell pepper, yellow, diced (1 cup)

- Tomatoes, un-drained, diced (14 ½ ounces)

Directions:

1. Fill a slow cooker with the turkey.

2. Meanwhile, place the beans in a large mixing bowl. Add the tomatoes, bell pepper, basil, and black pep-

per. Stir to combine.

3. Pour the bean mixture over the slow cooker turkey pieces. Cover and cook on low for four to six hours.

4. Transfer the cooked turkey onto individual plates. Smother with the bean mixture on top and garnish with basil leaves before serving.

5. Enjoy.

Turkey Spaghetti

Ingredients:

- Spaghetti, uncooked, broken up into 1/3-portions, cooked (8 ounces)

- Scallions, chopped (1/2 cup)

- Black pepper, freshly ground (1/8 teaspoon)

- Pimentos, canned, drained, sliced (1/4 cup)

- Flour, all purpose (3 tablespoons)

- Milk, skim, fat free (1/2 cup)

- Parmesan cheese, grated (3 ½ tablespoons)

- Margarine, reduced calorie (1 tablespoon)

- Button mushrooms, sliced (8 ounces)

- Garlic powder (1/4 teaspoon)

- Chicken broth, fat free (1 cup)

- Turkey breasts, skinless, boneless, cooked, cubed (1/2 pound)

- Cooking wine, sherry (2 tablespoons)

Directions:

1. Heat a large saucepan on medium-high before adding the margarine. Once hot and melted, stir in the mushrooms and scallions. Cook for about five minutes or until tender.

2. Place the flour in a large bowl. Add the pepper and garlic powder; stir to combine. Pour in the milk and broth, then whisk until well-blended.

3. Stir the flour mixture into the saucepan. Stirring fre-

quently, cook for about ten minutes or until the mixture boils and starts thickening.

4. Stir in the pimentos, turkey, and sherry. Cook for about two minutes or until the entire mixture is heated through.

5. Add the cooked spaghetti as well as the cheese. Gently toss to combine, making sure the spaghetti is evenly coated.

6. Serve and enjoy.

Turkey Tacos

Ingredients:

- Taco seasoning mix, dry (1 ¼ ounces)

- Turkey breasts, boneless, skinless (1 pound)

- Chicken broth, low sodium (1 cup)

Directions:

1. Pour the chicken broth in a large bowl. Add the taco seasoning and stir to combine.

2. Fill a slow cooker with the turkey breasts.

3. Add the broth mixture to the slow cooker, ensuring the turkey pieces are evenly covered.

4. Secure the slow cooker lid and allow the turkey to cook for six to eight hours on low heat.

5. Uncover and shred the turkey meat with two forks.

6. Cover again to cook on low for another half hour.

7. Serve as is, on top of your favorite salad, or stuffed into tacos.

8. Enjoy.

Wonderfully Succulent Turkey

Ingredients:

- Bread crumbs, Italian, whole wheat (1 ¼ cups

- Turkey breasts, boneless, skinless (3 pounds)

- Mayonnaise, light (1/2 cup)

Directions:

1. Set the oven to 425 degrees to preheat.

2. Brush all sides of the turkey with the light mayonnaise.

3. Pour the breadcrumbs all over the turkey, pressing lightly to ensure they adhere well.

4. Line a baking pan with foil. Add the coated turkey and place in the oven.

5. Bake for about forty to forty-five minutes or until the internal temperature of the meat reaches 165 degrees.

6. Serve immediately.

9 - Pork & Beef Recipes

Beefy Brown Rice and Black Bean Casserole

Ingredients:

- Swiss cheese, low fat, shredded (2 cups)

- Vegetable broth, low sodium (1 cup)

- Ground beef (1 pound)

- Black beans, drained (15 ounces)

- Onion, diced (1/3 cup)

- Cumin (1/2 teaspoon)

- Carrots, shredded (1/3 cup)

- Brown rice (1/3 cup)

- Olive oil, extra virgin (1 tablespoon)

- Zucchini, medium, sliced thinly (1 piece)

- Mushrooms, sliced (1/2 cup)

- Cayenne pepper (1/4 teaspoon)

- Green chilies, diced (4 ounces)

Directions:

1. Pour the vegetable broth into a large pot. Add the rice and stir, then allow the mixture to boil. Turn heat down to low before covering the pot and letting the rice mixture simmer for about forty-five minutes or until tender.

2. Meanwhile, set the oven at 350 degrees to preheat.

3. Use cooking spray (nonstick) to mist a casserole dish (large) until well-greased. Set aside.

4. Heat a large skillet on medium before adding in the olive oil. Stir in the onions and cook for two minutes or until tender and fragrant.

5. Add the seasonings as well as zucchini, mushrooms, and ground beef into the pan. Stir to combine and cook for another two to three minutes or until the zucchini is lightly caramelized and the entire mixture is heated through. Turn off the heat and set aside.

6. Transfer the cooked rice into a large bowl. Add the beef mixture as well as the beans, carrots, Swiss cheese (1 cup), and chilies. Toss to combine, then pour into the greased casserole dish.

7. Top with the remaining Swiss cheese (1 cup), then cover loosely with foil. Place in the oven to bake for half an hour.

8. Remove the dish from the oven. Uncover and return to the oven to bake for another ten minutes or until the surface is lightly browned.

9. Serve immediately.

Delicious Asian Style Pork Tenderloin

Ingredients:

- Brown sugar (1/3 cup)

- Mustard, dry (1 tablespoon)

- Garlic cloves, minced (4 pieces)

- Lemon juice, freshly squeezed (2 tablespoons)

- Pepper, freshly cracked (1 ½ teaspoons)

- Soy sauce, light (1/3 cup)

- Worcestershire sauce (2 tablespoons)

- Rice vinegar (2 tablespoons)

- Ginger (1 tablespoon)

- Pork tenderloin (2 pounds)

Directions:

1. Fill a large plastic bag (freezer-safe) with all the ingredients, except the pork tenderloin.

2. Toss the bag contents until well-combined.

3. Add the pork tenderloin and gently rub with the marinade.

4. Seal the bag and place in the refrigerator to marinate overnight.

5. Remove the bag from the refrigerator; place in the oven, preheated at 375 degrees), to bake for thirty to

forty minutes. (Alternatively, cook on low in the slow cooker for four to six hours.)

6. Pour into a serving bowl and serve immediately.

Easy Chili

Ingredients:

- Onion, chopped (1/2 cup)

- Jalapeno peppers, seeded, chopped (1/2 teaspoon)

- Sugar (1 teaspoon)

- Kidney beans, canned, rinsed, drained (4 cups)

- Cornmeal (2 tablespoons)

- Tomatoes, large (2 pieces)

- Celery, chopped (1 cup)

- Chili powder (1 ½ tablespoons)

- Water (as needed)

Directions:

1. Heat a soup pot on medium. Add the onion and ground beef, then sauté for two to three minutes or until the onion turns translucent and the meat is browned and cooked.

2. Drain the beef mixture before adding the celery, chili powder, sugar, kidney beans, and tomatoes. Stir to combine, then cover to cook for about ten minutes.

3. Stir in water and cornmeal. Allow the mixture to cook for ten to fifteen more minutes or until all the flavors are well-blended.

4. Transfer the chili into individual bowls (warmed). Top with jalapeno peppers before serving right away.

5. Enjoy.

Faux Fried Pork Tenderloin

Ingredients:

- Paprika (1/8 teaspoon)

- Soup mix, onion, dry (1 tablespoon)

- Bran cereal (1/3 cup)

- Salt, kosher (1/4 teaspoon)

- Buttermilk, reduced fat (1/3 cup)

- Pork tenderloin, raw, 1 1/4-inches each (10 pieces)

- Breadcrumbs, panko (1/3 cup)

Directions:

1. Pour the buttermilk into a large Ziploc bag. Add the paprika and combine well before adding in the chicken. Make sure the chicken is completely coated. Seal and place in the refrigerator for a minimum of one hour.

2. Set the oven at 375 degrees to preheat. Meanwhile, use cooking spray to coat a baking sheet (large).

3. Pour the cereal into the blender. Process until ground to a breadcrumb-texture. Transfer into a large mixing bowl. Add the onion soup mix as well as panko bread-crumbs. Stir to combine.

4. Take the chicken pieces out of the buttermilk bag and dredge in the breadcrumb mixture. Arrange on the prepped baking sheet and place in the preheated oven.

5. Bake for about ten minutes before flipping to cook on the other side for another ten minutes or until crispy and completely cooked. .

6. Serve and enjoy.

Pork Tenderloin and Apple Cider Curry

Ingredients:

- Curry powder (1 ½ tablespoons)

- Apple, tart, peeled, seeded, sliced into one inch cubes (1 piece)

- Yellow onions, medium, chopped (2 cups)

- Cornstarch (1 tablespoon)

- Pork tenderloin, sliced into 6 portions (16 ounces)

- Olive oil, extra virgin (1 tablespoon)

- Apple cider, divided (2 cups)

Directions:

1. Rub the curry powder onto all surfaces of the pork tenderloin; let sit for fifteen minutes.

2. Meanwhile, heat a large skillet (heavy bottomed) on medium-high before adding the olive oil. Add the seasoned pork tenderloin and cook for five minutes on each side or until browned and cooked through. Transfer onto a plate and let sit to cool.

3. Fill the same skillet with the onions. Stir and cook for two minutes or until golden and softened. Pour in the apple cider (1 ½ cups); stir to combine and turn the heat down to medium-low. Allow the mixture to simmer until reduced to ½ its original volume.

4. Stir in the cornstarch, remaining apple cider (1/2 cup), and the apple cubes. Let the mixture simmer for two minutes or until thickened, then add the cooked pork tenderloin. Let the mixture simmer again for five minutes before removing from the heat.

5. Transfer the pork tenderloin onto a platter. Drench with the sauce.

6. Serve and enjoy.

Stir-Fried Ginger Beef

Ingredients:

- Water chestnuts, sliced (8 ounces)

- Garlic cloves, medium (2 pieces)

- Cornstarch (1 tablespoon)

- Bell pepper, medium, green/ red/ yellow, sliced into strips (1/2 piece)

- Hoisin sauce (2 ounces)

- Red pepper flakes, crushed (1/4 teaspoon)

- Bok choy stalks, medium, sliced into half inch strips (2 pieces)

- Flank steak, sliced into quarter-inch strips (1 pound)

- Beef broth, fat free (6 ounces)

- Canola oil (1 teaspoon)

- Broccoli florets (3 ounces)

- Brown rice, instant (1/2 cup)

Directions:

1. Place the steak in a large bowl. Add the ginger and garlic, then toss to combine. Let sit while you work on the rice.

2. Follow package directions in cooking the rice.

3. Meanwhile, fill a medium bowl with the broth. Add the cornstarch, soy sauce, and hoisin sauce. Stir to combine, making sure the cornstarch is completely dissolved. Set aside.

4. Heat a large skillet on medium-high. Add the oil, then stir in the red pepper flakes. Add the steak and cook for two to three minutes on each side or until browned and cooked through. Remove from heat and set aside.

5. Add the bell pepper, carrot, and broccoli to the same skillet. Cook for about two to three minutes or until nicely crisp yet tender.

6. Add the water chestnuts and bok choy; stir and cook for two more minutes or until the bok choy is crisp but still tender.

7. Create a well in the skillet mixture's center, then fill with the broth. Stirring occasionally, let the north cook for one to two minutes or until thickened.

8. Stir in the beef and cook for one to two minutes or until heated through.

9. Pour your stir-fried ginger beef over rice and serve right away.

10. Enjoy.

Slow Cooker Beef with Brown Rice

Ingredients:

- Onion, large, diced (1 piece)

- Greek yogurt, plain (1 ½ cups)

- Paprika (1/2 tablespoon)

- Bay leaves (2 pieces)

- Ginger, fresh, minced (2 tablespoons)

- Garam masala (2 tablespoons)

- Black pepper, freshly ground (3/4 teaspoon)

- Cilantro, fresh, chopped (a handful)

- Ground beef (3 pounds)

- Garlic cloves, minced (4 pieces)

- Tomato puree (29 ounces)

- Olive oil, extra virgin (2 tablespoons)

- Cumin (1 tablespoon)

- Cinnamon (3/4 teaspoon)

- Cayenne pepper (2 teaspoons)

- Brown rice, cooked

Directions:

1. Fill a large bowl with all the ingredients, except for the chicken and bay leaves.

2. Stir to combine before adding the chicken. Stir again to coat the chicken thoroughly.

3. Transfer the chicken mixture to the slow cooker. Top with the bay leaves before covering.

4. Cook for four hours on high or eight hours on low.

5. After discarding the bay leaves, top with the cilantro and serve over brown rice.

Tart 'n Sweet Pork

Ingredients:

- Pineapple chunks, canned, unsweetened (15 ounces)

- Table salt (1/2 teaspoon)

- Brown rice, cooked (3 cups)

- Splenda (1/4 cup)

- Green peppers, medium, sliced (2 pieces)

- Pork tenderloin lean, sliced thinly into strips (1 pound)

- Water (1/2 cup)

- Onion, small, sliced (1 piece)

- Wine vinegar (1/3 cup)

- Cornstarch (2 tablespoons)

- Soy sauce, low sodium (1 tablespoon)

Directions:

1. Heat a large skillet (nonstick) on medium-high after generously coating with cooking spray.

2. Stir in the pork strips; cook for about four to five minutes or until golden brown. Once done, transfer onto a plate and let sit. Discard any remaining skillet fat.

3. Meanwhile, drain the pineapple chunks, setting aside the juice in a medium bowl. Add the water, soy sauce, vinegar, cornstarch, sugar, and salt. Stir to combine before adding to the skillet. Allow the mixture to cook for about two minutes or until thickened.

4. Stir in the cooked pork strips and reduce heat to low. Cook for another thirty minutes or until the meat has tenderized.

5. Stir in the drained pineapple chunks as well as onion and peppers. Allow the mixture to cook for five more minutes or until heated through.

6. Pour on top of cooked brown rice.

7. Serve and enjoy.

10 - Veggie Recipes

Baked Broccoli and Eggs

Ingredients:

- Margarine, light (4 ounces)

- Broccoli, frozen, thawed, chopped (10 ounces)

- Pimento, jarred, chopped (4 ounces)

- Flour (6 tablespoons)

- Black pepper, freshly ground (1 dash)

- Mushrooms, sliced, fresh (1/2 cup)

- Eggs, large (6 pieces)

- Cheddar cheese, low fat (1/2 pound)

- Cottage cheese, nonfat (2 pounds)

- Salt (1 teaspoon)

- Paprika (1 dash)

Directions:

1. Set the oven to 350 degrees to preheat.

2. Meanwhile, place the eggs, broccoli, and all other ingredients in a large bowl. Stir to combine.

3. Use cooking spray to coat the sides and bottom of a casserole dish (2-quart).

4. Fill the prepped dish with the broccoli-egg mixture, making sure to spread it evenly.

5. Bake in the oven for one hour and thirty minutes.

6. Serve immediately.

Black Bean and Pumpkin Soup

Ingredients:

- Onion, medium, chopped (1 piece)

- Black pepper, freshly ground (1/2 teaspoon)

- Pumpkin puree, canned (16 ounces)

- Cumin, ground (1 tablespoon)

- Tomatoes, canned, diced (1 cup)

- Olive oil, extra virgin (2 tablespoons)

- Garlic cloves, minced (4 pieces)

- Chili powder (1 teaspoon)

- Black beans, canned, rinsed, drained (30 ounces)

- Beef broth, low sodium (2 cups)

Directions:

1. Heat a soup kettle on medium after filling with the oil.

2. Add the garlic, onions, pepper, chili powder, and cumin. Stir and cook for about two to three minutes or until soft and fragrant.

3. Add the broth as well as pumpkin, tomatoes, and black beans. Stir to combine.

4. Allow the mixture to simmer, uncovered, for twenty-five minutes or until thickened to your desired consistency.

5. Remove from heat and process the black bean and pumpkin soup with an immersion blender.

6. Serve and enjoy.

Broccoli and Tofu Quiche

Ingredients:

- Salt (1/4 teaspoon)

- Mushrooms, chopped (1/4 pound)

- Pickled plum/ white miso paste (1 tablespoon)

- Yellow onion, chopped (1 piece)

- Sesame tahini (2 tablespoons)

- Bulgur wheat, uncooked (1/2 cup)

- Sesame oil (1 tablespoon)

- Broccoli, chopped (1/2 pound)

- Tofu (1 ½ pounds)

- Tamari (1 tablespoon)

Directions:

1. Set the oven at 350 degrees to preheat.

2. Fill a small pot with water (1 cup) and heat on medium. Bring to a boil before adding in the bulgur and salt. Stir to combine and allow the mixture to boil again.

3. Reduce heat to low and cover to cook for about fifteen minutes. Meanwhile, grease a pie pan (9-inch) with a little oil.

4. Pour the cooked bulgur into the pie pan, pressing lightly to spread it evenly at the bottom. Place in the oven to bake for about twelve minutes or until crusty on top. Let stand to cool.

5. Heat a large skillet (nonstick) on medium-high before adding the onions. Stir in the mushrooms and broccoli and cook for two minutes. Cover and immediately remove from heat.

6. Meanwhile, fill the food processor with the tofu. Add the tamari, tahini, and umeboshi paste. Process until

well-combined and smooth, then pour into a large bowl. Add the cooked veggies and gently toss until evenly coated.

7. Transfer the veggie mixture onto the crusted bulgur. Bake in the oven for about half an hour. Once done, let stand on a wire rack.

8. After ten minutes, slice into 6 portions and serve immediately.

Cheese-Filled Acorn Squash

Ingredients:

- Tofu, firm (1 pound)

- Basil (1 teaspoon)

- Black pepper, freshly ground (1 pinch)

- Onion, chopped finely (1 teaspoon)

- Garlic powder (1 teaspoon)

- Cheddar cheese, reduced fat, shredded (1 cup)

- Acorn squash, halved, seeded (2 pieces)

- Celery, diced (1 cup)

- Mushrooms, fresh, sliced (1 cup)

- Oregano (1 teaspoon)

- Salt (1/8 teaspoon)

- Tomato sauce (8 ounces)

Directions:

1. Set the oven at 350 degrees to preheat.

2. Arrange the acorn squash pieces, with their cut-sides facing down, at the bottom of a glass dish.

3. Place in the microwave oven and cook for about twenty minutes or until softened. Set aside.

4. Heat a saucepan (nonstick) on medium, then add the tofu (sliced into cubes). Cook until browned before stirring in the onion and celery. Cook for two minutes or until the onion is translucent.

5. Add the mushrooms. Stir to combine and cook for an additional two to three minutes. Pour in the tomato sauce as well as the dry seasonings.

6. Give everything a good stir, then spoon equal portions of the mixture inside the acorn squash pieces.

7. Cover and place in the oven to cook for about fifteen minutes. Uncover and top with the cheese before returning to the oven. Cook for five more minutes or until the cheese is melted and bubbling.

8. Serve immediately.

Cheesy Spinach Bake

Ingredients:

- Eggs, whole (2 pieces)

- Parmesan cheese (1/2 cup)

- Cottage cheese, fat-free/ low fat (2 cups)

- Spinach, frozen, thawed, drained (10 ounces)

Directions:

1. Set the oven to 350 degrees to preheat. Meanwhile, line a baking pan (8x8) with parchment paper.

2. Place all ingredients in a large bowl. Stir to combine.

3. Pour the cheesy spinach mixture into the prepped pan.

4. Place in the oven to bake for twenty to thirty minutes or until the cheese on top is bubbling.

5. Remove from the oven and allow to cool for five minutes.

6. Serve sprinkled with garlic, salt, and pepper.

7. Enjoy.

Mushroom and Wild Rice Soup

Ingredients:

- Onion, white, chopped (1/2 piece)

- White wine (1/2 cup) OR chicken broth, fat free, low sodium (1/2 cup)

- Thyme, dried (1/4 teaspoon)

- Carrots, chopped (1/4 cup)

- Milk, half and half, fat free (1 cup)

- Wild rice, cooked (1 cup)

- Olive oil, extra virgin (1 tablespoon)

- Celery, chopped (1/4 cup)

- White mushrooms, fresh, sliced (1 ½ cups)

- Chicken broth, fat free, low sodium (2 ½ cups)

- Flour (2 tablespoons)

- Black pepper, freshly ground (1/2 teaspoon)

Directions:

1. Heat a stock pot on medium, then add the olive oil.

2. Stir in the chopped onion as well as carrots and celery. Cook for two to three minutes or until tender and fragrant.

3. Pour in the chicken broth and white wine. Add the mushrooms as well, then stir to combine. Cover and allow the mixture to get heated through.

4. Meanwhile, place the flour in a large bowl. Add the milk, pepper, and thyme; stir to combine. Add the cooked rice and toss until well-combined.

5. Transfer the rice mixture into the vegetable pot. Stir well before cooking on medium until bubbly and thickened.

6. Serve immediately.

Mushroom and Zucchini Boats

Ingredients:

- Mushrooms, button, sliced (1 pound)

- Tomato, large, diced (1 piece)

- Pepper, freshly cracked (1/4 teaspoon)

- Egg, beaten (1 piece)

- Breadcrumbs, whole wheat, seasoned (1/4 cup)

- Mozzarella cheese, low fat, shredded (1 cup)

- Zucchini, medium (4 pieces)

- Onion, chopped (1/2 cup)

- Mushrooms, sliced (1/2 pound)

- Spaghetti sauce (3/4 cup)

- Salt, kosher (1/4 teaspoon)

Directions:

1. Set the oven at 350 degrees to preheat.

2. Slice the zucchini into lengthwise halves, then chop a thin slice off the zucchini bottoms so they can sit flat. Remove the pulp and place in a large bowl; set aside.

3. Meanwhile, arrange the empty quarter-inch shells at the bottom of a microwave-safe dish (3-quart, un-greased). Cover before placing in the microwave; heat on high for three minutes or until the shells are crisp and tender. Drain well before setting aside on a plate.

4. Heat a large skillet on medium. Add the onion and

mushrooms, stir well, and cook for five minutes or until tender. Turn off the heat and set aside.

5. To the bowl containing the zucchini pulp, add the breadcrumbs, cheese (1/2 cup), spaghetti sauce, tomato, pepper, salt, beaten egg, and the cooked mushrooms. Toss gently to combine.

6. Fill each zucchini shell with the mushroom mixture (1/4 cup), then top with the rest of the cheese. Place in the preheated oven to bake for about twenty minutes or until browned on top.

7. Serve and enjoy.

Nom Nom Veggie Burger

Ingredients:

- Mustard (1 tablespoon)

- Hamburger bun, whole wheat (1 piece)

- Ketchup, homemade (1 tablespoon)

- Burger, mozzarella flavored (1 piece)

- Mayonnaise, homemade (1 tablespoon)

- Tomato slices

- Lettuce leaves

- Onion slices

Directions:

1. Follow package directions in cooking the mozzarella flavored burger.

2. Top the hamburger bun with the cooked veggie burger.

3. Finish the burger by topping with the homemade mayonnaise and ketchup, lettuce leaves, and tomato and onion slices.

4. Serve and enjoy.

Quick Spinach Frittata

Ingredients:

- Onion, medium chopped (1 piece)

- Eggs, whole (2 pieces)

- Nutmeg (1/8 teaspoon)

- Cheddar cheese, reduced fat, shredded (1 ½ cups)

- Cayenne pepper (1/4 teaspoon)

- Vegetable oil (2 teaspoons)

- Spinach, frozen, thawed, drained, chopped (10 ounces)

- Egg whites (4 pieces)

- Cottage cheese, reduced fat (1/3 cup)

- Salt (1/8 teaspoon)

Directions:

1. Set the oven at 375 degrees to preheat. Meanwhile, use oil spray (vegetable) to coat a pie pan (9-inch).

2. Heat a medium-size skillet over medium-high heat. Add the oil; once heated through, stir in the onion. Cook for about five minutes or until the onion is

softened.

3. Stir in the spinach. Let the mixture cook for another three minutes before setting aside.

4. Meanwhile, fill the bottom of the pie pan with cheese before topping with the spinach mixture.

5. Place the whole eggs in a large bowl. Add the egg whites as well as cottage cheese, nutmeg, salt, and cayenne pepper. Stir to combine and pour on top of the cheese and spinach layers.

6. Place in the oven to bake for thirty to thirty-five minutes or until set.

7. Let cool for five minutes before slicing into wedges.

8. Serve and enjoy.

Vegetarian Chili and Cheese

Ingredients:

- Olive oil, extra virgin (2 teaspoons)

- Tomatoes, canned, diced (14 ½ ounces) OR fresh (2

cups)

- Red kidney beans, canned, rinsed (30 ounces)

- Onion, chopped (1 cup)

- Chili powder (2 tablespoons)

- Cheddar cheese, low fat, shredded (1 cup)

- Garlic cloves (2 pieces)

- Green bell pepper, large, diced (1 piece)

- Mushrooms, sliced (1/2 pound)

- Tomato sauce (8 ounces)

- Zucchini, medium, sliced thinly (1 piece)

- Corn, frozen (10 ounces)

Directions:

1. Heat a large skillet on medium-high before adding the olive oil.

2. Stir in the onions as well as mushrooms and green

pepper. Cook for two to three minutes or until tender and fragrant.

3. Pour in the tomato sauce along with the chili powder and diced tomatoes. Stir well before allowing the mixture to boil.

4. Reduce heat to low and then stir in the kidney beans and zucchini. Simmer the mixture for about ten to fifteen minutes.

5. Stir in the cheddar cheese (1/2 cup) and frozen corn before letting the mixture simmer for another ten to fifteen minutes.

6. Top with the remaining cheddar cheese and serve right away.

11 - Snacks & Treats Recipes

Apple and Squash Bake

Ingredients:

- Apples, medium, peeled, cored, sliced thinly into wedges (2 pieces)

- Flour, all purpose (1 tablespoon)

- Salt (1/3 teaspoon)

- Butternut squash, medium, peeled, sliced into ¾-inch cubed pieces (1 piece)

- Splenda (1 tablespoon)

- Butter, melted (1/4 cup)

- Cinnamon, ground (2 teaspoons)

Directions:

1. Fill a casserole dish with the apples and squash. Stir together until combined.

2. Place the rest of the ingredients in a medium bowl.

Stir to combine and pour on top of the apple-squash mixture. Give everything a good stir before covering with foil.

3. Place in the oven to bake for about fifty minutes or until tender.

4. Remove the foil and cook for another ten minutes or until crispy on top.

5. Serve and enjoy.

Cheesy Fluffs

Ingredients:

- Whipped topping, sugar-free (8 ounces)

- Cottage cheese, fat-free (48 ounces)

- Gelatin, sugar-free, flavored (6 ounces)

Directions:

1. Place the whipped topping, cottage cheese and gelatin in a large bowl.

2. Stir until well-combined.

3. Serve topped with blueberries and enjoy.

Chicken and Cheese Quiche

Ingredients:

- Chicken breast, grilled, sliced into one-inch cubes (6 ounces)

- Eggs, large (3 pieces)

- Oregano (1/8 teaspoon)

- Swiss cheese, low fat, sliced into cubes (4 ounces)

- Mozzarella cheese, low fat, shredded (10 ounces)

- Milk, skim (1 cup)

Directions:

1. Set the oven to 400 degrees to preheat.

2. Meanwhile, use cooking spray (nonstick) to lightly coat a pie pan. Fill with the chicken breast and Swiss

cheese cubes, making sure they evenly cover the bottom of the pan. Top with the shredded mozzarella before sprinkling with oregano.

3. Pour the skim milk and eggs into a large bowl. Whip until well-combined and smooth, then pour on top of the chicken-cheese mixture.

4. Place in the oven to bake for about forty minutes or until lightly brown on top.

5. Remove from the oven and allow to slightly cool.

6. Serve and enjoy right away.

Deliciously Spicy Deviled Eggs

Ingredients:

- Egg whites, hard boiled (6 pieces)

- Egg yolks, hard boiled (3 pieces)

- Dill (1/2 teaspoon)

- Salt (1/8 teaspoon)

- Horseradish sauce, creamy (2 tablespoons) OR Greek yogurt, plain (2 tablespoons)

- Mustard, spicy (1/4 teaspoon)

- Paprika (1/4 teaspoon)

- Black pepper, freshly ground (1/4 teaspoon)

Directions:

1. Remove the peel off each egg before slicing into lengthwise halves.

2. Pour 3 egg yolks into a large bowl (reserve the egg whites and the remaining three yolks).

3. Add the Greek yogurt/ horseradish sauce as well as salt, dill, and mustard. Whisk to combine.

4. Fill each halved egg white with the egg filling, then sprinkle with the paprika and pepper.

5. Serve and enjoy.

Dreamy Pumpkin Mousse

Ingredients:

- Vanilla pudding, fat-free (4 ounces)

- Milk, skim (1/2 cup)

- Splenda (1/4 teaspoon)

- Ginger, minced (1/4 teaspoon)

- Allspice (1/4 teaspoon)

- Clove (1/4 teaspoon)

- Nutmeg (1/4 teaspoon)

- Pumpkin, canned (15 ounces)

- Whipped topping, sugar-free (2 cups)

- Cinnamon (1 teaspoon)

Directions:

1. Place all ingredients in a large bowl.

2. Whisk until well-combined and evenly smooth.

3. Serve and enjoy.

Egg Enchilada

Ingredients:

- Black pepper, freshly ground (1/4 teaspoon)

- Salsa (2 tablespoons)

- Greek yogurt, fat-free, plain (2 tablespoons)

- Egg, whole (1 piece)

- Egg white (1 piece)

- Tofu (1 ounce)

- Cheese, Mexican blend, shredded (1 tablespoon)

Directions:

1. Place the egg as well as egg white in a medium bowl. Whip together until scrambled.

2. Heat a skillet (nonstick) on medium after coating its

bottom with cooking spray.

3. Add the scrambled egg mixture and spread into a round shape. Cook without stirring for one to two minutes or until firm on the edges. Sprinkle on salt and black pepper before flipping to the other side. Cook for another one to two minutes or until cooked through.

4. Slide the cooked egg onto a plate. Add the tofu and cheese, then roll up.

5. Serve your egg enchilada topped with Greek yogurt and salsa.

6. Enjoy right away.

French Toast Sandwiches

Ingredients:

- Ricotta cheese, fat-free (1/2 cup)

- Egg whites (3 pieces)

- Pumpkin pie spice (1/4 teaspoon)

- Bread slices, reduced calorie (4 pieces)

- Stevia (2 packets)

- Salt (1/4 teaspoon)

- Vanilla (1/4 teaspoon)

Directions:

1. Top each slice of bread with equal portions of the ricotta. Sprinkle inthe sugar substitute (1 packet per bread slice). Top with the remaining bread slices. Set aside.

2. Meanwhile, place the egg whites in a medium bowl. Beat until combined, then stir in the salt, vanilla, and pumpkin pie spice.

3. Heat a nonstick skillet (coated with cooking spray) on medium. Coat each sandwich in the egg white mixture, then add to the heated skillet. Cook for five minutes or until browned on each side.

4. Serve and enjoy.

Power Pancakes

Ingredients:

- Baking soda (1/2 teaspoon)

- Canola oil (1/2 tablespoon)

- Flour, all-purpose (1/3 cup)

- Cottage cheese, low fat (1 cup)

- Eggs, beaten lightly (3 pieces)

Directions:

1. Fill a medium bowl with the baking soda and flour. Stir to combine and set aside.

2. Fill a large bowl with the rest of the ingredients. Stir to combine before adding the flour mixture. Keep stirring until the flour mixture is incorporated into the cheese mixture.

3. Meanwhile, heat a large skillet on medium after lightly coating with cooking spray. Add the prepared

batter in batches and cook for two minutes or until bubbling on the surface. Flip to cook the top sides for one minute or until browned.

4. Pour in some syrup (low-calorie) and serve right away.

5. Enjoy.

Turkey-Stuffed Cabbage Rolls

Ingredients:

- Brown rice (1/3 cup)

- Ground turkey, 93-percent lean (1 pound)

- Tomato sauce (2 cups)

- Onion, medium, diced (1/2 piece)

- Oregano/ Italian seasoning (2 teaspoons)

- Cabbage head, w/ individual leaves removed (1 piece)

- Olive oil, extra virgin (1 teaspoon)

- Carrots, medium, diced (2 pieces)

- Garlic powder (2 teaspoons)

Directions:

1. Set the oven at 350 degrees to preheat.

2. After washing the cabbage leaves, blanch for half a minute and set aside in a medium bowl.

3. Follow package directions in cooking the rice.

4. In the meantime, heat a large skillet on medium before adding the olive oil. Stir in the onions as well as carrots; cook for three to four minutes or until softened and caramelized.

5. Stir in the turkey and cook for ten minutes or until browned and cooked through.

6. Stir in the seasonings as well as powders, then add the cooked rice. Toss gently to combine.

7. Fill the center of each cabbage leaf with half a cup of the turkey-rice mixture. Roll up and seal the edges

before placing in the baking dish, making sure their seams are facing down.

8. Smother the cabbage rolls with tomato sauce and place in the preheated oven. Bake for about thirty-five to forty-five minutes or until done.

9. Remove from the oven and let stand to cool.

10. Serve after five to ten minutes.

Book 1 - Gastric Sleeve Cookbook

Effortless Guide To Survive And Thrive Post-Surgery (Weight Loss Surgery Tips, Bariatric, Roux-en-Y, Sleeve Diet, Emotional Support)

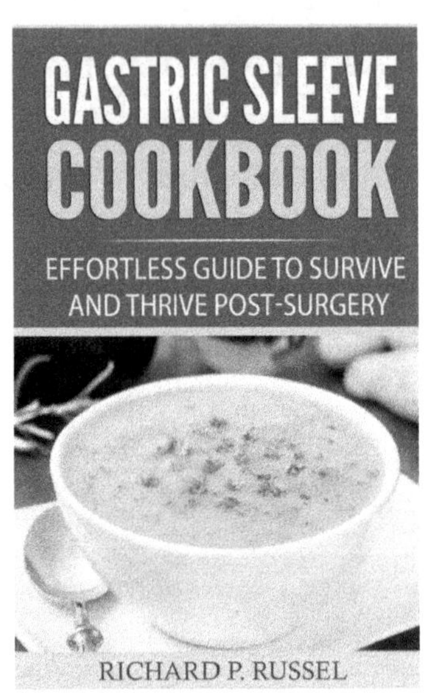

1 - Introduction

I want to thank you and congratulate you for buying this book.

This book contains proven steps and strategies on how to understand what you will go through after undergoing gastric sleeve surgery. It helps to prepare you for the emotional, psychological, and physical challenges that you will face as you journey towards losing weight. It also sheds light on the common nutrition complications and how you can cope with them.

This book explains the diet phases that you have to religiously follow before and after the surgery. It provides ample recipes that you can prepare after you have fully recovered and are ready to adapt to a healthier lifestyle with stricter food choices. Remember that the surgery is a life-altering procedure. It prompts you to lead a healthier lifestyle in order to lose weight and maintain your ideal figure.

Thanks again for buying this book, I hope you enjoy it!

2 - An Overview of the Gastric Sleeve Surgery

Bariatric surgery is an effective weight loss technique, which also lowers your risk of various health ailments associated with obesity. It works in two ways: malabsorption and restriction. Malabsorption happens as a result of the bypass of a portion of your small intestine.

As a result, your body will get a minimal amount of nutrients and calories. Restriction happens as the number of calories that you eat becomes limited. The operation works by physically limiting the amount of food that your stomach can take.

There are 4 common types of weight-loss surgery:

Laparoscopic adjustable gastric banding

During the surgery, a band that has an inflatable balloon is fixed in the upper area of the stomach. It becomes a small stomach pouch located at the upper part of the band with a small opening to the stomach. A port is also inserted beneath the skin of the abdomen, which is connected to the band via a tube.

The balloon can be inflated or deflated by removing the fluid through the port. This makes it possible to adjust the size of the band. The process limits the amount of food that the stomach can carry. It makes you feel full sooner but your body is still able to absorb the right amount of nutrients and calories.

Biliopancreatic diversion with duodenal switch

The process removes a large part of the stomach. The surgeon retains the duodenum or the first part of the small intestine and the valve responsible for the food discharge to the small intestine. The duodenal switch is performed by closing the center part of the small intestine and the last part is attached to the duodenum.

The part of the intestine that is separated is then reattached to the rear portion of the intestine. This allows the biliopancreatic diversion or when that portion of the intestine receives the flow of pancreatic digestive juices and bile.

The changes result in the limited nutrients and calories absorption since the food bypasses most parts of the small intestine. This factor along with the smaller size of your stomach will result in weight loss.

Roux-en-Y gastric bypass

In this process, a small pouch is created at the upper portion of the stomach. The pouch is the only area where food can go through. This means that you will have a greater limit of the amount of food and drinks that you can comfortably take at a time. The small intestine is trimmed near the bottom part of the stomach and connected to the pouch.

As a result, the main portion of the stomach continues to process digestive juices as the food travels from the pouch to the small intestine. The surgeon makes connections so that the digestive juices also flow through the small intestine. This setup limits the calories and nutrients absorbed by the body.

Sleeve gastrectomy

Similar to the biliopancreatic diversion, this process separates and removes a part of the stomach from the body. The remaining portion of the tummy is transformed into a structure that looks like a tube. Since the stomach is smaller, it can only hold a limited amount of food.

The process also causes a limited production of ghrelin, an appetite-regulating hormone. This makes you crave less for food. Unlike the biliopancreatic diversion though, this process doesn't limit the absorption of the nutrients and calories.

3 - More about the Gastric Sleeve Surgery

Gastric sleeve or sleeve gastrectomy is becoming the most preferred method among the other weight loss surgeries. It is faster and has a lower risk of complications. Other than these, gastric sleeve offers the following advantages over the other methods:

1. You will have a reduced appetite and less cravings for food.

2. The procedure is laparoscopic, which is less invasive since it only requires small abdominal incisions.

3. It doesn't involve a bypass. The digestive system will not experience rerouting, unlike the other methods. After the process, the stomach will continue to function as usual but since it is smaller, you will feel full sooner.

4. There are patients who don't qualify for gastric bypass surgery that are allowed to undergo gastric sleeve surgery. These are the patients who have a history or are suffering from certain health problems

that include Crohn's disease and anemia.

5. It takes a shorter period to finish the procedure. The surgery takes an hour or so, which makes the amount of time under anesthesia shorter. The hospital stay is also shorter at around 1 to 2 days.

6. It has fewer complications than the other weight loss surgeries.

7. The process is irreversible but if you experience a stall in weight loss, it can be converted to a gastric by-pass 6 to 18 months after the procedure.

8. Nothing needs to be realigned after the process since there are no foreign objects inserted into your body. This also means fewer follow-up visits to your doctor.

9. It only restricts the quantity of food that you can take, but you will still be allowed to eat healthy prepared food after the operation.

10. The feeling of fullness is comfortable and normal, unlike the feeling of pain or obstruction that is associated with the adjustable band surgery.

Aside from all these advantages, more people are choosing the gastric sleeve method because it is the least expensive method among the other weight loss procedures.

4 - How do you qualify for a gastric sleeve procedure?

Adult and young adult patients who have a Body Mass Index (BMI) of 30 or more are the ideal candidates for gastric sleeve surgery. This is also recommended for obese individuals who have tried all techniques to lose weight but failed, especially the patients who are at a high risk of health problems and death.

Here are the other factors to consider in order to qualify for the procedure:

- You have a stable mental health condition.

- You have been obese for over 5 years and have tried the traditional weight loss methods but repeatedly failed.

- You are not addicted to alcohol or drugs and you don't smoke.

- For women, you must be about 100 or more pounds overweight. For men, you have to be 80 or more pounds overweight.

4 - HOW DO YOU QUALIFY FOR A GASTRIC SLEEVE PROCEDURE?

- This procedure is life-changing. You have to commit to long-term lifestyle changes in order to continue losing weight and maintain the weight that you have already lost.

5 - What are the risks and disadvantages that the procedure entails?

The complications and risks that you may suffer from after the procedure are minimal as compared to the side effects of the other weight loss surgeries. Here are the complications that you can expect following a gastric sleeve procedure:

- You will experience minor side effects immediately after the surgery. They include swelling, bleeding, bruising, and pain. For many of those who have undergone the procedure, these side effects naturally disappear several days up to a few weeks after the surgery.

- Only a few patients have complained of more severe side effects such as leaking or internal bleeding, too much pain, gastritis, and bloating in the abdominal area. There are also a small number of patients who develop pneumonia, vomiting, and infection. If you experience any of these severe side effects, make sure that you have yourself checked immediately by a doctor.

- Weight loss is gradual and may not be as great as compared to the more invasive forms of weight-loss surgeries.

- Less than 1 percent of the gastric sleeve patients experience blood clots, which can be fatal.

- It is important that you change your lifestyle after the procedure. You have to strictly follow the diet restrictions or else, the sleeve will stretch out and you will gain weight.

6 - What is the next step to do if you are interested to undergo gastric sleeve surgery?

Ask around or research for the qualified medical team that is an expert in the field and near your area. Make an appointment and consult with the doctor to learn what other things you need to prepare for before the operation.

Make sure that you know or have jotted down the following details:

- Your medical history including anesthesia complications. You will also be asked about the health history of your parents and siblings.

- Make a list of the drugs over-the-counter or prescription-type, food or herbal supplements, and vitamins that you regularly take.

- Ask your doctor about the available payment methods. If you are insured, be sure to ask what portion of the process is covered by the insurance.

- Ask all your concerns and anything that will make it

easier for you to prepare for the operation.

You have to prepare your body for the drastic changes that you will implement after the surgery. Exercise more often. You can start by walking for several minutes at the start of your day.

If you are a smoker, it is best to quit as soon as you have set your mind to undergo the procedure. Smoking makes the lungs more sensitive during the process. This makes you at a high risk of pneumonia. This will also make the healing process slow because the effects of smoking make the blood vessels narrow, which restricts your blood flow.

Due to the risks involved with smokers, many surgeons do not operate on patients who are smokers. Aside from the interview, they will require you to undergo tests to check the nicotine levels in your system before approving your request.

You must also expect drastic changes in your diet before and after the procedure. To help you cope easily with these changes, start implementing the following diet preparation tips:

6 - WHAT IS THE NEXT STEP TO DO IF YOU ARE IN-TERESTED TO UNDERGO GASTRIC SLEEVE SURGERY?

1. Avoid drinking high sugar drinks until you are no longer craving for them. Avoid drinking carbonated drinks because they tend to make you feel full faster and could potentially stretch your stomach after the operation.

2. Learn how to prepare your meals in different ways aside from frying. You have to start cutting down your intake of fried food.

3. Start getting used to drinking fluids in between meals and not with meals. This is something that you will practice for a lifetime after the procedure.

4. Start using a sugar substitute instead of table sugar.

5. Start cutting down your alcohol intake. Alcohol contains empty calories that have no place in your diet after the operation.

6. You have to start chewing your food thoroughly. Decrease the portion sizes of each meal and eat three meals a day.

7. Eat healthily and focus on proteins.

8. Gather a support group. Research about online forums and groups that you can join to discuss the situation with before and after the surgery. You also need to talk to your friends and family about the situation. You need a strong support to help you in many ways, especially in the emotional aspect of the process.

7 - What should you expect weeks and days before you undergo the operation?

Before the operation, you've already had a number of consultations with your surgeon. You will be asked to undergo different exams and lab tests. At this point, you must already have adapted to the drinking and eating restrictions.

Two weeks prior the surgery, your surgeon will require you to follow a special diet. This will prepare your body for the procedure and increase the chance for a successful outcome. Many of those who suffer from severe obesity have enlarged livers. This condition will make the surgery difficult to perform. The diet aims to reduce the size of the liver and the amount of fat in the abdominal area.

The directives about the diet must come from your surgeon. Here's a peek at what the diet looks like to give you an idea of what you need to prepare yourself for:

- Limit your calorie intake to 1000 to 1200 each day.

- Your diet must contain low fat and low carbohydrate.

- You are required to take 6 to 8 glasses of fluids each day in order to prevent dehydration. Aside from water, you can take other sugar-free, non-carbonated, low-calorie, and caffeine-free liquids.

- Your diet must contain lots of protein. You may also be instructed to take protein supplements. This is important to protect your muscle tissues and help your body recover faster after the operation.

- You will be asked to take one protein shake for breakfast and lunch, and a lean protein and salad for dinner.

Protein supplements can be bought as powders or ready-to-drink. Here are some insightful tips for making your own protein shake:

- Add the protein supplement to plain non-fat yogurt. Mix well until combined.

- If your system cannot tolerate dairy, you can use plain soy milk or fat-free Lactaid milk.

- Pour skim milk into ice cube molders. Put into a

blender once firm and process until slushy.

- Make a protein shake latte by adding a teaspoon of decaffeinated instant coffee.

Here are the other food items that are typically included in this diet 2 weeks before the procedure:

- Vegetable juice or V8

- Soup and broth without any solid particle

- Extremely thin cream of wheat or cream of rice

- Sugar-free beverages

- Protein and meal replacement shakes

At this point, you can no longer take your liquids with meals. Take them 30 minutes before and after eating. Always remember to sip them slowly.

If you want to eat solid food, get the approval of your doctor first. If he/she agrees, you can have a couple of servings of lean meat and vegetables.

What if instead of losing weight, you incur a significant increase in your weight during this period? Your doctor will adjust the date of your surgery up to the time that you have lost 10 to 15 pounds prior to the operation.

Your doctor will only allow you to take protein shakes a day before the surgery. After 5 PM, you need to consume clear liquids, such as tea, Jell-O, ginger ale, broth, and water. You cannot take anything after midnight so that your stomach will be empty by the time of the operation.

Before the surgery, ask your doctor for the kind of support that they offer throughout the recovery process. List out the hospital and your medical team's emergency contact numbers so that you would know who to turn to when something strange happens while you are recovering from home.

Arrange for someone to accompany you to the hospital. If you live alone, ask someone to stay with you at home even for several days after the procedure. Your movements will be limited for the first few days during the recovery period. The least that you want to happen is to get stressed. You will need a lot of assistance in doing cooking and certain hygienic tasks.

7 - WHAT SHOULD YOU EXPECT WEEKS AND DAYS BEFORE YOU UNDERGO THE OPERATION?

Make sure that you have the following items at home before the operation:

- Canned broth

- Doctor-approved protein shakes and meal replacements

- Sugar substitutes and sugar-free flavors

- Soups with smooth texture

- No-sugar-added pudding, popsicles, and Jell-O

- Doctor-approved vitamins and minerals

- Small food containers, freezer bags, and kitchen tools

- Blender or food processor

8 - What should you expect after the operation?

Sleeve gastrectomy reduces the size of your stomach by up to 90 percent. Do not expect that you will lose weight immediately after the surgery. It is a process that requires your cooperation. There is a diet plan that is classified according to stages to help you in the healing process.

The size of your stomach a couple of hours after the surgery can hold about 2 ounces of nourishment. How will the first few hours after the operation be like?

- A nurse will monitor whatever pain you are feeling. The medication will pass through an IV and the amount of medication will depend on your initial level of pain. Prepare yourself because it can really get painful and it worsens through the hours.

- When you are already fully awake, a nurse will encourage and assist you to walk. This will help improve the functions of your urinary tract and gastrointestinal tract that slowed down after the operation. Walking will lower your risk of post-operation complications. This helps in maintaining your normal breathing function and encourages the movement of oxygen throughout your system.

- After the surgery, you will be allowed small sips of liquid or ice chips to stay hydrated. Your IV will be removed once your stomach can tolerate sufficient liquids to keep you hydrated.

- If there are no complications and the doctor sees you fit to go home, you will be allowed to do so on the second day of your hospital stay.

9 - The 5 Stages of a Gastric Sleeve Diet

You will follow a 5-stage diet plan upon coming home. In order to help your body recover faster, eat food rich in nutrients and vitamins. After you have fully recovered, your diet will be more restricted and nutritionally-balanced.

Here are the general rules on what to do in order to avoid complications and other problems after the procedure:

1. Make it a habit of eating your food and drinking fluids in a slow manner. Consume each meal for at least 30 minutes. Eating and drinking too quickly may cause nausea and vomiting.

2. Chew your food thoroughly and until it already has a liquid consistency before swallowing.

3. Do not drink fluids while eating. This is necessary to avoid the expansion of the stomach due to bloating. Drink your fluids 30 to 60 minutes before and after meals.

4. Follow the daily amount of fluids and food that your doctor recommends. It is important that you don't

gain weight during the recovery stage. If you will get bigger, this might lead to a rupture that will jeopardize the process.

5. Avoid dehydration by following the recommended amount of fluids according to the diet phase that you are in. Dehydration can lead to vomiting and diarrhea.

6. Avoid high caloric food with minimal nutrients and those with high sugar content. These foods will make it more difficult for you to lose weight.

10 - The 5 Stages of a Gastric Sleeve Diet

Clear Fluids (1 to 2 days after the operation)

This will begin upon waking up in the hospital after the operation. Your fluid intake is limited to 30 cubic centimeters of water every hour. Keep a fluid record sheet to monitor how much you have already taken.

For the first day, drink 15 ml of clear fluids every 15 minutes. Aside from water, you can also consume broth, tea, no-sugar-added Jell-O, and diluted fruit juice. You won't get dehydrated despite the restricted amount of fluid because you will still be on an IV at this point.

On your second day, you will follow the same diet in the hospital upon coming home. Slowly sip 30 ml of clear fluid every 15 minutes.

11 - Liquid Diet (Weeks 1 and 2 following the procedure)

This diet will begin on the third day after the operation. You need to drink up to 4 cups of water and take at least 70 grams of protein per day. You will also begin taking the chewable vitamins and supplements recommended by your health team.

What are you allowed to take during this phase?

Beverages

- Sugar-free clear fluids

- Water

Soups (smooth, strained, and free of lumps)

- Butternut soup

- Potato soup

- Tomato soup

Protein sources

- Skim milk or 1 percent milk

- Lactose-free milk

- Plain or natural soy drink

- Protein powder

- Protein shakes

- No sugar added yogurt

- Cottage cheese

Vegetable and Fruit

- Tomato juice

- Unsweetened apple juice

Starch and grain

- Cream of wheat

- Oatmeal (with less than 10 grams of sugar)

Keep in touch with your health team. Observe how your body responds to the new diet scheme. If you experience nausea, vomiting, and severe abdominal pain, go back to the first diet plan for the next 24 hours. If the problems continue for more than 12 hours, call your doctor and ask for an advice.

Recommended Multivitamins (liquid and chewable):

1. Multivitamin. Take 1 tablet twice a day of a chewable supplement rich in vitamins and minerals.

2. Calcium sources. Take the following chewable tablets twice each day: Caltrate 600 + D, Calcium Citrate + D, and Viactiv Calcium + D. Each tablet must contain at least 600 mg of calcium and 400 IU of vitamin D.

3. Vitamin B12 sublingual. Take a tablet each day by putting it under your tongue until it dissolves.

Always consult your nutritionist before buying any vitamins and supplements. It is important that you those that meet your nutritional requirements depending on the diet stage that you are in.

Sample meal plan for a day:

Breakfast: Vanilla-Strawberry shake and 1 small pack of no sugar added low-fat yogurt

Snack: A cup of protein shake

Lunch: 1/4 cup of low-fat cottage cheese, 1/4 cup of plain low-fat yogurt, and 1/4 cup tomato juice

Snack: Half a cup of protein shake

Dinner: 1/4 cup of applesauce and 1/4 cup of strained cream of chicken soup with protein powder

Snack: Half a cup of protein shake

Here's a sample meal plan for those who are lactose intolerant or developed this complication after the procedure:

Breakfast: 1/4 cup of tomato juice, 1/2 cup of strained potato soup with 1 tablespoon of protein powder, oatmeal, and peach chai protein shake.

Oatmeal is prepared by putting 1/2 cup of oats in a bowl and mixing it with 1 cup of lactose-free milk.

To prepare the peach chai protein shake, put the following ingredients in a blender: 1/3 cup of unsweetened soy beverage, 1/2 fresh peach, 1/3 cup of brewed Chai tea, 1 scoop of vanilla protein powder, 1/4 teaspoon of pumpkin pie spice, and 2 ice cubes. Process until smooth.

Lunch: 1/2 cup of strained potato soup with 1 tablespoon of unflavored protein powder.

Snack: Protein water

To make protein water, mix 1 scoop of unflavored protein powder, 1 cup of water, and 1 packet of crystal light in a container. Cover and shake well until combined.

Dinner: 1/4 cup of applesauce, 1/2 cup of strained vegetable soup with 1 tablespoon of protein powder.

Snack: 1/4 cup cream of wheat

12 - Pureed Diet (Weeks 3 and 4 after the operation)

At this stage, you will reintroduce your stomach to food that you used to eat before the operation but in soft and pureed forms. The process should be gradual. Remember to always take it easy and keenly observe how your body reacts to what you are eating. If you experience any pain or if you vomit after eating, go back to the previous diet. Let 24 hours pass before going back to this diet.

Vomiting is likely to happen at this point. Take note of the food that made you feel sick. Remove it from your menu for the next 2 to 3 weeks. You can still eat all the food items from the past diet phases though. Continue to take chewable vitamins and the mineral and protein supplements.

You must also remember to take up to 1.5 liters of calorie-free liquids each day. To make it easier to meet the daily protein requirement of 70 grams, you can add unflavored protein powder to your food and consume 2 protein shakes each day.

What are you allowed to take during this phase?

Vegetables and fruits

- Tomato juice

- Unsweetened applesauce

- Cooked or canned pureed vegetables and fruits

Starch and grains

- Cream of wheat

- Cold cereal soaked in milk

- Oatmeal with less than 10 grams of sugar

- Soda crackers

- Melba toast

All kinds of pureed soups

Beverages

- Water

- Decaffeinated tea or coffee

- Juice diluted in water

- Low-fat vegetable or meat broth

- Sugar-free clear fluids

Desserts

- No sugar added Jell-O

- No sugar added ice cream

- No sugar added pudding

Protein sources

- Protein shakes

- Skim milk or 1 percent milk

- Lactose-free milk

- Protein powder

- Ricotta cheese

- Cream cheese

- Cottage cheese

- No sugar added yogurt

- Moist and mashed fish

- Plain or natural soy beverage

- Pureed meat, including chicken, beef, and pork

- Hummus

- Soft poached egg

How to poach an egg:

Boil 2-inch deep of water in a small pan. Turn the heat to low once the water is boiling. Crack an egg into a bowl. Carefully lower the bowl into the water and let the egg slip out. Cook until done but soft.

Sample meal plan for a day:

Breakfast: 2 tablespoons of pureed fruit, 1/3 cup of cream of wheat mixed with 4 tablespoons of milk

Snack: A cup of protein shake

Lunch: 1 soft poached egg and 2 pieces of Melba toast

Snack: 1 small pack of no sugar added yogurt

Dinner: 4 tablespoons of mashed fish or pureed meat, 2 tablespoons of pureed carrots and 2 tablespoons of mashed
potato with 1 tablespoon of unflavored protein powder

Snack: A cup of protein shake

13 - Soft Diet (Weeks 5 to 9 after the procedure)

At this point, your daily protein requirement is 80 to 80 grams. Continue drinking protein shakes, unless your dietitian tells you otherwise. Continue taking your protein supplements. Start taking vitamins and mineral supplements in pill form.

In the beginning, break the pills into smaller pieces in order to avoid any discomfort. Increase your calorie-free fluid intake to 2 liters a day. It is also important that you slice your food into smaller pieces before you eat.

If you feel any discomfort, stop eating the food that caused the pain. Go back to the previous diet and try this phase again after a few days.

To keep your food moist and tender, it is best to prepare them using a slow cooker or a crackpot. Here's a list of the foods that you can reintroduce to your diet:

- Cereals with high fiber and low sugar

- Boiled or scrambled eggs, cooked with little or no fat

- All kinds of cheese, sliced into 1-inch pieces

- All soups

- Pita bread and tortilla wraps

- Well-toasted bread, thinly sliced

- Soft fruits, such as peeled mango, apple, and banana

- Diced or ground poultry or meat, cooked in chili, stew, or curry

- 1 tablespoon per serving of cashew butter, peanut butter, or almond butter

- Soft legumes cooked with sauce

Sample meal plan for a day:

Breakfast: 1/4 cup of ricotta cheese, 1/4 cup of no sugar added canned peaches (diced), and 1 tablespoon of bran flakes with a bit of cinnamon

Snack: Half a cup of protein shake

Lunch: 1/2 cup of bean soup, 1 cheese string, and 1 Melba toast

Snack: 1 small pack of no sugar added yogurt

Dinner: 2 tablespoons of well-cooked vegetables, 2 ounces of stewed chicken, and 1/4 cup of mashed potato

Snack: 1/4 whole wheat pita with ¼ cup of tuna and 2 teaspoons of light mayonnaise, 1/2 cup of protein shake

14 - Lifelong Healthy Eating

This is the start of your regular diet. This is a lifelong process and you have to stick to it in order to keep losing weight and maintain your ideal shape. You will gradually decrease the number of protein supplements that you are taking. Instead, you will consume more protein with the food that you eat. Avoid taking sweets, such as ice cream and cookies, fats, cheap calories, junk food, and high-calorie liquids.

More Tips to Make the Diet Work

1. Stop eating once your body tells you that it is full.

2. Avoid eating junk food and sweets. Eat solid food instead to relieve hunger and forget about your cravings.

3. If you feel hungry in between meals, drink instead of eating. You may only be thirsty and not hungry. You can also snack on any food items with no calories. Train yourself to eat only during meal times.

4. It is up to you to make the operation successful. You have to stick to the 5-stage diet plan during the recov-

ery period and change your diet for a lifetime. You cannot go back to your old ways before the surgery. The diet has to be teamed up with regular exercise and healthy lifestyle.

5. Pre-portion your meal by using a small plate. Always eat in a slow manner and chew your food well. Stop whenever you feel full even if you still haven't finished your meal. Refrigerate your food instead and reheat when it is time for the next meal.

6. Monitor your protein intake. If you haven't reached your daily protein goal of 60 to 80 grams when it is already night time, supplement by preparing and taking a protein shake.

15 - What are the foods rich in protein?

This list contains food that you can include in your diet to help you meet your daily protein requirement. The list includes how many grams of protein you can get per serving of each food item:

Milk and alternatives

- 1/3 cup of plain, flavored, low-fat, or regular yogurt – 4 grams

- 1/2 cup of 1 percent skim milk – 4 grams

- 1/2 cup of plain soy drink – 3 grams

- 1/3 cup of plain Greek yogurt – 8 grams

- 1/2 cup of 1 or 2 percent cottage cheese – 8 grams

- 1 slice of regular or processed cheese – 3 grams

- 2 tablespoons of skim milk powder – 5 grams

- 1-inch cube of light Mozzarella cheese – 7 grams

- 1-inch cube of regular Mozzarella cheese – 6 grams

- 1-inch cube of cheddar cheese – 7 grams

- 1/4 cup of part-skim or whole ricotta cheese – 7 grams

Chicken and meat

- 1/4 cup of chopped deli ham – 6 grams

- 1/4 cup of diced chicken – 10 grams

- 1/4 cup of diced beef steak or beef roast – 11 grams

- 1/4 cup of chopped deli turkey breast – 6 grams

- 1/4 cup of diced pork – 10 grams

- 1/4 cup of crumbled lean beef – 9 grams

- 1/4 cup of diced turkey – 10 grams

Fish

- 1/4 cup of chopped smoked salmon – 6 grams

- 1/4 cup of fresh or canned tuna – 10 grams

- 1/4 cup of shrimp – 8 grams

- 1/4 cup of canned or filet salmon – 9 grams

- 1/4 cup of scallops – 8 grams

- 1/4 cup any variety of flaked fish – 9 grams

Meat alternatives

- 1/4 cup of lentils – 5 grams

- 1/4 cup of baked canned beans – 3 grams

- 1/4 cup of kidney beans – 5 grams

- 1/4 cup of chickpeas – 4 grams

- 1/2 cup of chili – 9 grams

- 1 tablespoon of peanut butter – 4 grams

- 1/4 cup of soft tofu – 3 grams

- 1/2 cup of split pea or bean soup – 9 grams

- 1/4 cup of dry textured vegetable protein – 12 grams

- 1/4 cup of edamame – 6 grams

- 1/4 cup of hummus – 5 grams

- 1 egg white – 3 grams

- 1/4 cup of firm tofu – 5 grams

- 1 egg (whole) – 6 grams

- 1 egg yolk – 3 grams

- 1/3 cup of meatless ground meat – 10 grams

After you have achieved your weight loss goal in a span of 6 months to a year, your daily calorie requirement will increase to 1000 to 1200. Your lifelong diet will change not only with regards to what you eat but also on how you eat your food. Always remember to:

Avoid drinking fluids along with your meals. Drink 30 or 60 minutes before and after meals.

- Chew your food thoroughly and swallow only when it has a liquefied consistency.

- Eat a small portion of food at a time and stop eating once you already feel full.

- Avoid fast food, oily, and fatty food.

- Bring a healthy snack with you wherever you go in order to avoid the temptation to eat whatever is available when hunger strikes.

- Avoid high calorie and carbonated drinks.

Follow your doctor's advice when it comes to exercise. He/she will tell you once your body can handle the activity and the kinds of exercises you can do depending on the progress of your recovery.

16 - The Emotional Pitfalls and the Most Common Complications of the Surgery

No matter how determined you are to lose weight, there will always be emotional and psychological challenges once you have undergone the surgery. These challenges will depend on how long you have been obese.

Obesity is associated with lack of self-confidence, low self-esteem, and depression. You used to deal with these emotions by eating a lot. This is a habit that you have to overcome once you have decided to undergo the procedure but it won't be easy.

Weight loss surgery is a major operation that entails a lot of drastic changes in all aspects of your life. You can help yourself by staying fit physically and mentally. Find a doctor who can counsel you and your support groups, including your family and friends. This will help a lot, especially at times when you feel like giving up.

What are the most common emotional pitfalls that you may face after the operation?

Anxiety. After the surgery, you may get overwhelmed with the new social activities and new situations that you would want to try but too scared to proceed. It is okay to feel anxious, especially in the beginning. Ask support from people who care about you to talk and push you towards trying out new things. Consult and ask a therapy if your anxiety becomes too much to handle.

Insecurity. It will take time to remove your old image from your mind and accept that you are no longer the fat person that you considered normal. There will always be a feeling of insecurity with how you look and how other people see you even after you have lost a lot of weight.

Talk to people who have experienced the same thing. Hang out with groups composed of individuals who have undergone the same procedure.

Relationship changes. If you are in a relationship, open your mind that the changes will not only affect you but also your partner. It can either make good relationships better but can also make it worse. The improved physical appearance can result in a healthy intimacy and active sex life.

On the other hand, this can also make your partner feel insecure or jealous. Before the relationship turns sour, seek counseling as a couple and go through this together. You have to reassure your partner, and both of you need to be open about your feelings towards each other.

Depression. Not everything will be pretty after the surgery. You won't lose weight immediately after coming home from the hospital. The strict diet is not easy to follow. After the surgery, you will be faced with sagging skin here and there, especially when you are beginning to lose weight. Set your expectations right. Help yourself to deal with the changes and effects of the surgery as they happen.

When things and emotions get too much to handle, always ask emotional support from your family and friends. Never hesitate to go to your doctor when the emotional turmoil won't get away. Keep yourself busy with sports, hobbies, and other activities that will help in keeping your mind off

from the emotional and psychological setbacks of the surgery.

17 - Ways to Adjust Emotionally and Physically after the Surgery

Keep a diary or a journal. Write everything – your thoughts, struggles, the feeling of joy and accomplishments. Write everything down. Keep track of the food that you eat, the food that made you feel sick, activities that you have tried, and so on. You can always read your entries at times when you feel like giving up and turning to your old habits.

Writing about how you feel and what you are going through will help you to easily cope and adjust to the changes. This is your way to talk to yourself and understand your own emotions regarding the effects of the surgery.

Move on and adapt to the changes but do not forget what you have gone through that led you to undergo the procedure. It will make it easier for you to accept the new you if you will remember how it was before.

Ask for help whenever you feel like you need to. Do not keep your problems to yourself. Accept that you will need a lot of support from groups, from your loved ones, and counseling sessions with your doctor. By opening up and meeting people who have experienced the same things that you are going through, you will feel that you are not alone.

Do not be too hard on yourself. Set realistic goals and write them down in your diary. You can modify the goals depending on how your body is recovering from the operation.

Keep track of your body measurements. Take pictures of yourself to make it easier for you to monitor your physical changes. Keep your old clothes. Wearing them after you have achieved your ideal weight will give you a sense of fulfillment.

This will help you a lot, especially at times when you experience a weight loss plateau. This will serve as a visual reference to help you erase the image of your old self and remind you that you are losing weight.

Try different things. Experience and live life. Do not shy away from the new experiences and people that you meet.

Take your doctor's advice seriously. Follow his/her recommendations regarding the diet, exercises, and the supplements that you are taking. You need to take lots of rest to speed up the recovery process.

18 - The Most Common Complications of Gastric Sleeve Surgery

Most complications are likely to happen due to the changes in your digestive tract. The best that you can do to reduce your risk of having any of these is to stick to your diet and keep yourself fit. It is also important that you don't drink any alcoholic beverages for the first 6 months after the operation to avoid the risk of having an ulcer.

Dehydration

This common complication of the procedure is a signal that your body lacks fluid. The smaller size of your pouch makes it harder to drink sufficient liquid. How would you know that you are already dehydrated?

- You are constantly thirsty.

- Your urine is dark-colored and you urinate less often.

- Headache and dizziness

- Dry mouth, lips, skin, and eyes

- Feeling annoyed and tired

Make sure that you drink up to 6 cups of water each day to avoid getting dehydrated. You can also suck on ice chips and popsicles because they count as fluids, too. You can add flavors to your water to tweak its taste.

Infused ice cubes. Put an herb, a slice of fruit or a combination of these two in an ice cube tray. Pour boiling water to instantly release the flavors and aromatic compounds of the herbs. Leave to cool before freezing.

Cucumber and mint. Rinse the cucumber, thinly sliced, and put into a pitcher full of water. Add mint and put the pitcher in the fridge. The longer it stays in the fridge before you drink it, the more flavors the water will have. Add more water to reuse the flavors. Discard after 3 days and replace with new mint and cucumber slices.

Watermelon. Slice the fruit into cubes. Put them in a pitcher full of water. You can add mint if preferred. Refrigerate for a couple of hours before drinking.

Basil and blueberries. Rinse the basil and blueberries. Put the basil in a pitcher full of water. Crush the berries before mixing them with the water. Refrigerate before drinking.

Sugar-free lemonade and berries. Squeeze a couple of drops of sugar-free lemonade into a pitcher full of water. Grate the strawberries and add them to the water. Add a few slices of lemon. Refrigerate before consuming.

Hypoglycemia

The symptoms of hypoglycemia or low blood sugar include dizziness, hunger, and cold and clammy skin. These symptoms typically show up after eating foods that are high in sugar, but they naturally go away after some hours. Here are the ways to prevent this kind of complication:

- Eat balanced meals and always eat on time.

- Make sure that your meals and snacks are filled with protein.

- Take carbs that are high in fiber and low in sugar.

Have a blood glucose meter handy at home to make it easier for you to monitor your blood sugar levels. The levels must not go lower than 4 millimoles per liter, or else you must take precaution and perform the following actions:

1. Consume 15 grams of fast-acting sugar. You can take any of the following: 3 dextrose tablets, 1 tablespoon of sugar mixed with 2 tablespoons of water, 3/4 cup of juice, and 1 tablespoon of honey.

2. Lay down to rest for at least 15 minutes.

3. Check your blood sugar and repeat the first 2 steps if the result is still not higher than 4 millimoles per liter. Continue repeating the first 2 steps until the result reflects your goal.

4. Snack on items with protein and carbs, which include the following:

- Apple with peanut butter

- Hummus and carrots

- Greek yogurt with fruit slices

- Melba toast with cheese

Diarrhea

Your body is trying to adjust to the effects of the procedure. It is also trying to cope with the changes in its digestive mechanism. Diarrhea can also be a sign of a dumping syndrome. If you experience this complication, make sure that you avoid the following food:

- Milk products

- Caffeinated drinks

- Fatty food

- Food with high sugar alcohol content

Eat food items with soluble fiber, which include applesauce, oatmeal, and bananas. You can also take a dietitian-approved fiber supplement. This complication is not alarming but consult with your doctor if it lasts for more than 3 days.

Food intolerance

There are certain foods that you may find hard to digest at first, which include the following:

- Dried fruit

- Rice

- Skins of fresh fruit

- Pasta

- Fried and fatty foods

- Chicken or red meat

- Milk and milk substitutes

- Bread

- Beverages and sugary products

- Chocolate and candy

These food may likely cause pain or pressure in your stomach area. Keep track of the food that made you feel that way. Consult it with your dietitian so that he/she can find the better alternative.

Dumping Syndrome

This happens when the food that you have taken travels fast from the stomach to the small intestine. As a result, you will experience the following symptoms:

- Heart palpitation

- Explosive diarrhea

- Dizziness

- Stomach pain and cramping

- Upset stomach

- Sweating

- Nausea

- Flushing

The signs can show up an hour or two after eating, but they can also happen sooner. Make sure that you don't drink fluids with your meals. This complication is likely experienced from eating any of the following:

- Sweetened yogurt

- Frozen yogurt

- Ice cream

- Gelato

- Frozen or canned fruit in syrup

- Sorbet

- Popsicles

- Regular pudding or Jell-O

- Undiluted fruit juices

- Candied or dried fruit

- Chocolate milk

- Honey

- Sweetened or sugar-coated cereal

- Cookies

- Milkshakes

- Pastries

- Muffins

- Chocolate

- Sweetened sauces

- Regular soft drinks

- Brown or white sugar

- Deep-fried food

Lactose intolerance

It is common to develop lactose intolerance after the procedure even if you were not like this before. It happens when the body doesn't produce sufficient enzymes to break down the sugar from lactose and milk products. The signs of this complication include the following:

- Diarrhea

- Bloating and gas

- Stomach pain and cramping

Try the following steps to deal with the problem:

- Consume lactose-free milk products.

- Eat yogurt of cheese instead of drinking milk.

- Take a liquid or chewable enzyme supplement before taking or eating milk products.

19 - Gastric Sleeve Appetizer Recipes

Here are the appetizer recipes that you can try and serve starting from the phase 5 of the diet and for the rest of your life.

Bacon Wrapped Chicken with Jalapeno

Yield: 30 pieces

Ingredients:

- 1 tablespoon each of onion powder, garlic powder, and freshly ground black pepper

- 1 onion, sliced into 30 strips

- 15 jalapeno peppers, halved and seeds removed

- 1 pound chicken breasts, skinless and boneless

- 1 pound bacon, sliced

- 2 teaspoon seasoned salt

- 1 teaspoon paprika

- Blue cheese salad dressing

Directions:

1. Slice the meat into 30 pieces strips.

2. Put together the salt, pepper, paprika, onion powder, and garlic powder in a Ziploc bag. Add the meat strips, seal the bag and shake. Put 1 chicken strip and 1 onion strip in each jalapeno half. Wrap with bacon.

3. Grill until the chicken is cooked and the bacon is crisp. This will take around 20 to 30 minutes. Turn once.

4. Serve the grilled bacon wrapped chicken with jalapeno with the dressing.

Deviled Eggs with Avocado

Yield: 1 dozen

Ingredients:

- 1/4 cup olive oil mayonnaise

- 5 slices bacon (center-cut), fried and crumbled

- 1 tablespoon each red onion (finely diced) and Dijon mustard

- Sea salt and paprika to taste

- 6 eggs, hard-boiled and peeled

- Parsley sprigs

Directions:

1. Slice the eggs in half. Scoop the yolks and put them in a bowl. Add the mustard and mayonnaise to the yolks. Mix and stir in the bacon, salt, and avocado.

2. Put a tablespoon of the mixture to each half of the egg white. Sprinkle paprika on top and garnish with parsley sprig. Loosely cover with foil and chill before serving.

Spinach Artichoke Dip

Yield: 16 servings

Ingredients:

- 1 10-ounce package frozen spinach, thawed, chopped,

and drained

- 5 bacon slices (center-cut), fried and crumbled

- 2 garlic cloves, minced

- 1/3 cup olive oil mayonnaise

- Cooking spray

- 1 teaspoon Herbes de Provence

- 2/3 cup Parmesan cheese, grated and divided

- 2 8-ounce packages cream cheese (with reduced-fat, room temperature

- 1 14-ounce can artichoke hearts, quartered, chopped, and drained

Directions:

1. In a bowl, put the cream cheese, mayonnaise, and garlic. Beat until mixed and creamy. Add the bacon, spinach, half of the cheese, and artichoke hearts, and stir.

2. Transfer the mixture to a greased baking dish. Sprinkle the rest of the cheese on top. Bake in a preheated oven at 350 degrees for 25 minutes.

This is best served with veggies and grain crackers.

Apple and Cranberry Salsa

Yield: 4 cups

Ingredients:

- 1 jalapeno pepper, seeds removed and sliced into strips

- 1 12-ounce package cranberries (fresh or frozen), rinsed and drained

- 1/4 cup fresh cilantro leaves

- 2 apples, cored and chunked

- 1/3 cup unsweetened applesauce

- 1/2 sweet red pepper, seeds removed and chunked

- 1 teaspoon grated lime peel

- 1/2 red onion, chunked

- 1 lime, juiced

- Sea salt and freshly ground black pepper to taste

- 1/2 cup sugar substitute

Directions:

1. Put all the ingredients in a blender. Pulse until chopped.

2. Transfer to a bowl, cover and refrigerate for an hour before serving.

Crispy Cheese

Yield: 8 crisps

Ingredients:

- 1/2 cup hard cheese, grated

Directions:

1. Put a tablespoonful of cheese on a baking sheet lined

with parchment paper. Press it into a thin circle. Repeat the process until you have used all the cheese. Leave a distance of about 2 inches in between the circles.

2. Bake in a preheated oven at 350 degrees for 15 minutes. Allow to cool before serving.

Spicy Pinto Bean Sauce

Yield: 2 cups

Ingredients:

- 1 teaspoon cumin

- 1 30-ounce can pinto beans, rinsed and drained

- 1/4 teaspoon each of sea salt, ground black pepper, and red pepper flakes

- 1/2 cup each of cream cheese (with reduced fat), water, and light sour cream

- 2 garlic cloves, minced

- 1 cup Mexican cheese blend, divided

- 1/2 teaspoon chili powder

Directions:

1. Put water, garlic, and beans in a food processor with a metal blade attachment. Pulse until almost mashed.

2. Transfer the mixture to a pan over medium heat. Season with salt, pepper, chili powder, cumin, and red pepper flakes. Stir in half a cup of cheese, sour cream, and cream cheese. Mix until combined.

3. Remove from heat once the mixture is heated through. Transfer to a heat-proof bowl. Sprinkle the rest of the cheese on top. Microwave for 40 seconds on a high setting.

This is best served with veggies and chips.

Shrimp with Cocktail Dipping

Yield: 10-12

Ingredients:

- 1/3 cup chili sauce

- 2 tablespoons prepared horseradish

- 2 teaspoons Old Bay seasoning

- 1 tablespoon fresh lemon juice

- 2/3 cup ketchup

- Chopped celery

- 1 teaspoon Worcestershire sauce

- 1/2 teaspoon lemon zest

- 2 pounds shrimp, peeled, deveined and cooked

Directions:

1. Put the cooked shrimp on a plate and lightly sprinkle with the seasoning.

2. In a bowl, mix the rest of the ingredients, except for the celery. Garnish the dipping with chopped celery and serve along with the shrimp.

Healthy White Bean Hummus

Yield: 1 1/2 cups

Ingredients:

- 2 garlic cloves, minced

- 1/4 cup each of water and extra-virgin olive oil

- 1/2 teaspoon sea salt

- 1 lemon, juiced

- 1/3 cup tahini

- 1 15-ounce can white beans, rinsed and drained

Directions:

1. Put all the ingredients in a food processor with a metal blade attachment. Process until smooth.

2. Transfer to a bowl. Serve along with veggies or pita chips.

You can opt to top the hummus with chopped artichoke

hearts or roasted bell peppers.

Mushroom Pizza

Yield: 12 mushrooms

Ingredients:

- 1/4 cup each of turkey pepperoni slices and grated Parmesan cheese

- 12 whole Crimini mushrooms

- Cooking spray

- 2 tablespoons each of sliced black olives and Italian-leaf parsley

- Garlic salt and ground black pepper to taste

- 1/8 of red onion, sliced

- 1/4 of green bell pepper, sliced

- 1/2 cup cream cheese (with reduced-fat), room temperature

- 1/2 teaspoon Italian seasoning

Directions:

1. Remove the stems of the mushrooms and wash with a damp cloth.

2. Put the rest of the ingredients in a food processor with a metal blade attachment. Process until combined with small chunks.

3. Put a spoonful of the mixture on each mushroom cap.

4. Arrange the stuffed mushrooms on a greased baking sheet. Bake in a preheated oven at 350 degrees for 20 minutes. Set the oven to broil and brown the tops of the mushrooms.

Thai Chicken Satay

Yield: 4-6 servings

Ingredients:

- 1 pound chicken tenders

- 1 lime, juiced

- 1 tablespoon each of fish sauce and soy sauce (low-sodium)

- 1/2 teaspoon chili garlic sauce

- 2 tablespoons sesame oil

For the peanut sauce

- 2 tablespoons peanut butter (smooth natural)

- 1 teaspoon brown sugar

- 1 tablespoon each of soy sauce (low-sodium), sesame oil, and fresh lime juice

- 2 tablespoons of light coconut milk

- 1/2 teaspoon chili garlic sauce

Directions:

1. In a shallow dish, combine the soy sauce, sesame oil, chili garlic sauce, fish sauce, and lime juice. Marinate the meat for 15 minutes.

2. Put 2 marinated chicken tenders on each skewer.

Wrap the end of the skewer with foil. Grill both sides of the meat until cooked.

3. Prepare the sauce by whisking the chili garlic sauce, peanut butter, lime juice, coconut milk, brown sugar, soy sauce, and sesame oil in a bowl.

4. Serve the grilled along with the sauce.

Stuffed Bell Peppers

Yield: up to 40 stuffed baby peppers

Ingredients:

- 20 baby bell peppers

- 2 garlic cloves, minced

- 1 teaspoon ground cumin

- 1/2 teaspoon sea salt

- 1/2 14.5-ounce can diced tomatoes (juice included)

- 1/2 15-ounce can black beans, rinsed and drained

- 1 4-ounce can mild diced green chilies (juice included)

- 1 tablespoon chili powder

- 1 1/2 cups Mexican cheese, shredded and divided

- 1/2 cup onion, chopped

- Fresh cilantro, chopped

- 1/2 pound ground turkey (99 percent fat-free)

Directions:

1. Cut each pepper in half and remove the top part, seeds, and membranes.

2. Cook turkey in a pan over medium-high flame until browned. Add garlic and onions, and cook for 4 minutes. Stir in the black beans, cumin, chilies, salt, tomatoes, and chili powder. Bring to a boil. Turn the heat to low. Simmer for 15 minutes before turning off the stove.

3. Allow the dish to slightly cool before adding a cup of

cheese and the cooked quinoa. Mix well.

4. Fill each pepper with a tablespoon of the mixture. Arrange the stuffed peppers on a baking tray and cover with foil. Bake in a preheated oven at 375 degrees for 30 minutes. Discard the foil. Sprinkle the rest of the cheese on top and bake for 5 more minutes.

5. Put chopped cilantro on top before serving.

Easy-to-Do 9-Layer Dip

Yield: 10-12 servings

Ingredients:

- 1 cup light sour cream

- 1 1.5-ounce pack taco seasoning

- 1 15-ounce can black beans, rinsed and drained

- 1 lime, juiced

- 1 cup grape tomatoes, halved

- 1 cup bottled mild salsa

- 2 tablespoons green onion, chopped

- 1 avocado, diced

- 1/2 cup fresh cilantro, chopped

- 1 1/2 cups grated cheddar cheese

- 1/2 cup red bell pepper, diced

Directions:

1. Transfer the beans to a plate. Mash them using a fork. Spread the mashed beans all over the plate. Sprinkle with the taco seasoning. Put sour cream on top of the beans. Gently spread but make sure that you do not mix salsa with the sour cream. Sprinkle cheese all over. Put the tomato halves on top. Pour lime juice all over the avocado before arranging them on top of the stack. Sprinkle the following in this order: green onions, red peppers, and cilantro.

2. Put in the fridge before serving.

Feta and Tomato Cheese Dip

Yield: 1 1/2 cups

Ingredients:

- 2 tablespoons pine nuts, toasted

- 2 tablespoons fresh basil, chopped

- 4 ounces sun-dried tomatoes (packed in oil), julienned

- 1/4 cup olive oil

- 4 garlic cloves, minced

- 4 ounces feta cheese, crumbled

Directions:

1. Put all the ingredients in a bowl. Toss to combine.

2. Serve the dip along with soft flatbread, sliced veggies, or pita chips.

Chicken Meatballs Southwestern Style

Yield: 24 small meatballs

Ingredients:

- 2 garlic cloves

- 3 green onions, trimmed

- 1 egg

- 1 1/2 pounds lean ground chicken

- 1 teaspoon cumin

- 1 jalapeño, seeds removed

- 1/4 cup fresh cilantro, chopped

- 1/2 red bell pepper, chunked

- A pinch oregano

- 1/4 cup breadcrumbs

- 1/4 teaspoon freshly ground black pepper

- 1/2 teaspoon sea salt

- Greek yogurt dressing

Directions:

1. Put the green onions, garlic, red bell pepper, cilantro, and jalapeño in a food processor with a metal blade attachment. Cover and pulse until minced.

2. Transfer the mixture to a bowl. Add the bread crumbs, ground chicken, salt, pepper, cumin, oregano, and egg. Mix thoroughly using your hands. Roll into small balls. Arrange the balls on a baking sheet lined with parchment paper. Bake in a pre-heated oven at 400 degrees for 15 minutes.

3. Serve the meatballs along with mashed avocado or Greek yogurt dressing.

20 - Gastric Sleeve Diet Breakfast Recipes

Spicy Egg Puff

Yield: 12 servings

Ingredients:

- 10 eggs

- 1/2 teaspoon salt

- 2 cups low-fat cottage cheese (2 percent)

- 4 cups Monterey Jack cheese, shredded

- 1/2 cup all-purpose flour

- 1 4-ounce can green chilies, chopped

- 1 teaspoon baking powder

Directions:

1. Beat the eggs in a bowl until fluffy.

2. In another bowl, mix the flour, salt, and baking

powder. Gradually add this to the beaten eggs. Mix until combined. Fold in the chilies and cheese.

3. Transfer the mixture to a greased baking dish. Bake in a preheated oven at 350 degrees for 40 minutes. Leave for 5 minutes before serving.

Banana-Strawberry Smoothie

Yield: 2 servings

Ingredients:

- 1/2 frozen banana

- 10 frozen strawberries

- 1/2 cup Greek yogurt (plain)

- 1 cup low-fat milk (1 percent) or light soy

- 1/2 tablespoon agave nectar

- 1 tablespoon ground flax meal

- 1 scoop whey protein powder (vanilla-flavored)

Directions:

1. Put all the ingredients in a blender. Process until smooth. Pour over 2 glasses and serve.

Cheesecake Parfait with Berries

Yield: 8

Ingredients:

- 4 ounces light cream cheese, softened

- 2 cups low-fat milk

- 1 cup sliced strawberries

- 1 cup fresh blueberries

- 1/4 teaspoon vanilla extract

- 2 tablespoons agave nectar

- 1/2 cup honey roasted almonds, chopped

- 1 4-serving package cheesecake instant pudding mix (sugar-free)

- 1 6-ounce pack strawberry cheesecake light yogurt

Directions:

1. Put the berries and agave nectar in a bowl. Mash some of the blueberries to get a little amount of juice out. Leave for 5 minutes but stir the mixture twice.

2. In another bowl, put the pudding mix, cream cheese, vanilla, yogurt, and milk. Beat for 3 minutes using an electric mixer set on medium-high speed. Cover the bowl and put in the fridge for 20 minutes.

3. Line up 8 parfait glasses. Put 2 tablespoons of the blueberry mixture in each glass. Add a tablespoonful of the cream cheese mixture and top with a table-spoon of chopped almonds. Serve immediately.

You can also cover the other glasses and put in the fridge for 8 hours before serving.

Spinach and Smoked Turkey Quiche

Yield: 12 servings

Ingredients:

- 1 cup fresh baby spinach leaves

- 1/8 tsp freshly ground black pepper

- 3/4 cup smoked turkey, cubed

- 1/2 cup fat-free half and half

- 1 teaspoon baking powder

- 3/4 cup shredded Swiss cheese, divided

- 1/2 cup chopped onion

- Cooking spray

- 2 eggs, plus 2 egg whites

- 1 cup low-fat cottage cheese (2 percent)

- 1/2 cup whole wheat pastry flour

- 1/4 cup shredded reduced-fat cheddar cheese

Directions:

1. Grease a nonstick skillet with cooking spray and place over medium-high heat. Put the meat, pepper, and

onion. Saute for 4 minutes.

2. Spread 1/4 cup of shredded Swiss cheese on a greased pie plate. Arrange the turkey mixture on top.

3. In a bowl, mix the rest of the Swiss cheese, cottage cheese, eggs and egg whites, half and half, and cheddar cheese. Whisk until combined.

4. Combine flour and baking powder in a bowl. Gradually add this to the egg mixture. Mix well. Pour this over the turkey mixture. Bake in a preheated oven at 350 degrees for 45 minutes.

Green Smoothie

Yield: 2 servings

Ingredients:

- 1 cup frozen peach chunks

- 1 cup frozen mango chunks

- 2 cups water

- 1 cup frozen pineapple chunks

- 2 tablespoons sugar substitute

- 2 cups fresh spinach, tightly packed

- 1/2 lemon, juiced

Directions:

1. Put water and spinach in a blender. Process for 2 minutes or until smooth. Add the peaches, mango, lemon juice, pineapple, and agave nectar. Process until smooth. Serve immediately.

Easy Breakfast Delight

Yield: 1 serving

Ingredients:

- 1 teaspoon chia seeds

- 1/2 apple, diced

- 1/4 cup almond milk or light vanilla soy

- 1 6-ounce pack Greek yogurt

- 1 tablespoon each of all or any of the following: toasted sunflower seeds, unsweetened shredded coconut, mini dark chocolate chips, toasted pistachio seeds, and toasted pumpkin seeds

Directions:

1. Transfer the yogurt to a bowl. Pour soy milk and top with all the ingredients. You can also use other toppings, such as chopped cashews, chopped walnuts, and toasted sliced almonds.

Crustless Vegetable Quiche

Yield: 8 servings

Ingredients:

- 3/4 cup asparagus spears, sliced

- Cooking spray

- 2 tablespoons green onion, sliced

- 1/2 green or red bell pepper, diced

- 1 tablespoon olive oil

- 2 garlic cloves, minced

- 2 cups fresh spinach leaves, packed

- 1 teaspoon ground thyme

- 1/4 cup cooked bacon, crumbled

- 4 ounces mushrooms, sliced

- 3 eggs, plus 3 egg whites

- 1/4 teaspoon freshly ground black pepper

- 1/2 teaspoon sea salt

- 1/4 cup Parmesan cheese, shredded

- 1/2 cup artichoke hearts (packed in water), chopped

- 1 1/4 cup cheddar cheese, shredded

- 3/4 cup fat-free half and half

Directions:

1. Heat oil in a pan over medium-high flame. Stir in the asparagus, artichoke hearts, garlic, green onion,

thyme, mushrooms, spinach, and bell pepper. Saute for 5 minutes. Add the crumbled bacon and season with salt and pepper. Leave to cool.

2. In a bowl, whisk the milk, salt, pepper, eggs, and egg whites.

3. Transfer the cooked vegetables to a greased pie pan. Sprinkle with shredded cheese. Pour the egg mixture and spread the shredded Parmesan cheese on top.

4. Bake in a preheated oven at 350 degrees for 45 minutes. Leave to cool for 10 minutes before slicing.

Cheesy Vegetarian Frittata

Yield: 6 servings

Ingredients:

- 1/2 zucchini, seeded and diced

- 1 tablespoon olive oil

- 2 ounces low-fat Mozzarella cheese, shredded

- 1/2 teaspoon dried ground oregano

- 4 ounces mushrooms, sliced

- 6 eggs, beaten

- 1/2 red or green, diced

- 2 ounces Parmesan cheese, shaved

- 2 ounces Feta cheese, crumbled

- 1 teaspoon seasoned salt

- 1/4 red onion, sliced

Directions:

1. Heat oil in an omelet pan over medium-high heat. Put the bell pepper, mushrooms, onion, and zucchini. Saute for 6 minutes. Turn the heat to low and add all the cheese. Leave the dish until the cheese melts. Put the eggs, oregano and seasoned salt. Cover the pan and cook for 12 minutes.

2. Remove the cover of the pan and put it in a preheated broiler. Broil for a couple of minutes or until the top part has browned.

3. Allow to cool a bit before slicing. Serve while warm.

Ricotta and Spinach Pie

Yield: 12 muffins or 1 whole pie

Ingredients:

- 1 garlic clove, minced

- 1/8 teaspoon ground nutmeg

- 1 tablespoon olive oil

- Salt and pepper to taste

- 1/2 cup onion, chopped

- 2 cups part-skim milk ricotta cheese

- 8 cups fresh spinach, chopped

- 1/4 cup Parmesan cheese, shredded

- 1 cup mozzarella cheese, shredded

- 1 pound turkey sausage (Italian-seasoned)

- 3/4 cup egg substitute

Directions:

1. Heat oil in a pan over medium-high flame. Cook the garlic and onions for 3 minutes. Stir in the spinach and cook for 5 minutes. Put the nutmeg, mix, and season with salt and pepper. Turn off the heat and leave to cool.

2. In a bowl, combine the egg substitute, parmesan, mozzarella, and ricotta cheese, and the sautéed spinach. Roll out the sausage on top and pour the filling. Bake in a preheated oven at 350 degrees for 30 minutes.

Banana-Apple Protein Smoothie

Yield: 2

Ingredients:

- 1/2 cup apple juice (unsweetened)

- 1 banana

- 1 tablespoon ground flax meal

- 1 tablespoon almond butter

- 2 teaspoon agave nectar

- 1/2 cup light Greek yogurt (vanilla)

Directions:

1. Put all the ingredients in a blender. Add 3 ice cubes. Process until smooth. Transfer to 2 glasses and serve.

21 - Gastric Sleeve Diet Salad Recipes

Broccoli and Chicken Salad

Yield: 8 servings

Ingredients:

- 1/2 cup red onion, diced

- 2 cups cooked chicken breasts, diced

- 1/2 cup carrot, shredded

- 3 cups broccoli florets, chopped

- 1/2 cup red grapes, halved

- 8 slices of bacon (center-cut), cooked and crumbled

- 1/2 cup cashews, toasted

For the dressing:

- 1/2 cup Greek yogurt (plain non-fat)

- 1/4 teaspoon sea salt

- 1/4 cup white wine vinegar

- 1/2 cup olive oil mayonnaise

- 2 teaspoons of sugar substitute

Directions:

1. Put the broccoli in a heat-proof bowl. Microwave for 3 minutes on a high setting. Immediately rinse under cold water and drain.

2. Put the broccoli in a bowl. Add the toasted cashews, carrot, onion, grapes, chicken, and bacon. Carefully mix to combine.

3. Mix the dressing in a bowl. Combine the vinegar, mayonnaise, sugar, salt, and Greek yogurt. Mix until creamy. Pour over the salad and toss to coat. Refrigerate before serving.

White and Black Bean Greek Salad

Yield: 6 servings

Ingredients:

- 1/3 cup red onion, chopped

- 4 ounces feta cheese (reduced-fat), crumbled

- 1/3 cup fresh mint leaves, chopped

- 1 15-ounce can white beans (reduced-sodium), drained and rinsed

- 1 15-ounce can black beans (reduced-sodium), drained and rinsed

- 1/2 cup cucumber, diced

For the dressing:

- 2 tablespoons agave nectar

- 3 tablespoons fresh lemon juice

- 1/2 teaspoon each of oregano leaves, celery seed, garlic powder, sea salt, and fresh ground black pepper

- 1/4 cup olive oil

Directions:

1. In a bowl, mix the cucumber, mint, beans, red onion, and feta.

2. Whip up all the ingredients for the dressing in another bowl. Pour over the salad and toss to coat.

3. Cover the bowl and chill for an hour before serving.

Chicken Caesar Salad

Yield: 6 servings

Ingredients:

- 1 cup canned garbanzo beans (reduced-sodium), drained and rinsed

- 2 cups romaine lettuce leaves, torn

- 1/2 cup cucumber, peeled and sliced

- 2 tablespoons green onions, sliced

- 1/2 pound chicken breasts (skinless and boneless), cooked and diced

- 2 ounces shaved Parmesan cheese and crumbled sun-dried tomato

- 1 cup cherry tomatoes, halved

- 1/2 cup light Caesar dressing

- 2 tablespoons fresh basil, chopped

Directions:

1. In a bowl, mix the garbanzo beans, lettuce, tomatoes, chicken, basil, green onions, and cucumber. Add the dressing and toss to combine. Top with cheese before serving.

Grape, Melon and Chicken Salad

Yield: 6 servings

Ingredients:

- 1/2 ripe cantaloupe, peeled and sliced into bite-size pieces

- 1/4 cup each of plain Greek yogurt, chopped cashews, and reduced-fat mayonnaise

- 1/2 cup each of halved red grapes and sliced celery

- 1/2 teaspoon salt

- 1/4 teaspoon fresh ground black pepper

- 1 orange, juiced

- 2 cups cooked chicken, cubed

Directions:

1. In a bowl, mix the celery, grapes, and chicken.

2. In another bowl, combine the orange juice, mayonnaise, salt, and yogurt. Pour this over the chicken mixture and toss to combine. Top with chopped cashews before serving.

Curry Chicken Salad with Coconut

Yield: 4

Ingredients:

- 1/4 cup shredded carrots

- 1/2 cup light coconut milk

- 2 tablespoons green onions, thinly sliced

- 2 tablespoons roasted peanuts, chopped

- 2 tablespoons fresh cilantro, chopped

- 4 green leaf lettuce leaves

- 1 tablespoon Thai green curry paste

- 1/4 cup unsweetened shredded coconut

- 1/2 cup red grapes, halved

- 1 1/4 cup chicken, cooked and shredded

Directions:

1. Put the curry paste and coconut milk in a bowl. Mix until smooth. Add the green onions, carrots, peanuts, chicken, coconut, grapes, and cilantro. Toss to combine.

2. Lay a lettuce leaf on a plate. Put 1/4 of the mixture. Roll the leaf and fold the ends.

You can serve this along with fresh fruit.

Spinach Salad with Chicken and Curry Dressing

Yield: 4-6 servings

Ingredients:

- 4 cups spinach leaves, sliced

- 1/4 cup almonds, sliced

- 1/4 cup green onion, sliced

- 2 teaspoons sugar substitute

- 1/2 cup diced celery

- 1 cup diced apple

- 1 cup cooked chicken, diced

For the creamy curry dressing:

- 1/4 cup Greek lemon yogurt

- 1/4 cup light olive oil mayonnaise

- 2 tablespoons water

- 3 tablespoons fresh lemon juice

- 1 teaspoon curry powder

- Sea salt and fresh ground black pepper to taste

- 1 teaspoon sugar substitute

Directions:

1. In a skillet over medium-high flame, combine the sugar substitute and almonds. Stir for 3 minutes. Transfer the cooked almonds to a waxed paper and arrange in a single layer. Allow to cool.

2. In a bowl, mix the chicken, spinach, green onion, celery, and apple.

3. Mix all the ingredients for the dressing. Toss with the apple and vegetable mixture. Top with sweetened almonds and serve.

Chicken Caprese Salad

Yield: 8 servings

Ingredients:

- 1 pound chicken breasts (skinless and boneless)

- 5 cups Romaine lettuce leaves, rinsed and torn

- 1 tablespoon olive oil

- 1 14-ounce can artichoke hearts, drained and quartered

- 2 cups cherry tomatoes, halved

- Sea salt and freshly ground pepper to taste

- 1 avocado, sliced

- 1/4 cup basil leaves, thinly sliced

- 1 cup mini mozzarella cheese balls, halved

For the dressing:

- 1 teaspoon sugar substitute

- 1/4 cup olive oil

- 1/4 cup balsamic vinegar

- 1 teaspoon sea salt

- 1 teaspoon minced garlic

- 1 teaspoon dried basil

Directions:

1. Put all the ingredients for the dressing in a bowl. Whisk to combine. Put 4 tablespoons of the mixture in a Ziploc bag. Add the chicken. Seal the bag and leave for 30 minutes.

2. Heat a tablespoon of oil in a pan over medium-high flame. Drain the marinade and put the chicken in the pan. Cook each side for 7 minutes. Turn off the heat and leave to rest for 10 minutes. Cut the meat into strips.

3. Arrange the lettuce on a platter. Add the tomatoes,

artichoke hearts, avocado slices, chicken, and mozzarella cheese. Put the basil strips on top. Drizzle with the rest of the dressing. You can opt to season the salad with salt and pepper.

Chicken Asian Salad

Yield: 8 servings

Ingredients:

- 4 chicken breasts, boneless, skinless and halved

- 2 teaspoons Chinese Five Spice powder

- 2 tablespoons sesame oil

- 2 tablespoons reduced-sodium soy sauce

- 1/2 teaspoon garlic powder

- 1 teaspoon sugar substitute

For the salad:

- 4 cups chopped cabbage

- 1/4 cup diced red onion

- 1/4 cup chopped peanuts

- 1/4 cup chopped fresh mint leaves

- 1/4 cup chopped fresh cilantro

- 1/2 cup diced red bell pepper

- 1/2 cup cucumber, diced, peeled, and seeded

- 1/2 cup shredded carrots

For the chili lime dressing:

- 2 tablespoons lime juice

- 2 tablespoons canola oil

- 1 tablespoon agave nectar

- 1 tablespoon chili garlic sauce

- Sea salt and freshly ground black pepper to taste

- 1/4 cup seasoned rice vinegar

Directions:

1. Put the following in a Ziploc bag: Five Spice powder, sugar substitute, soy sauce, garlic powder, and oil. Add the chicken and seal the bag. Leave for an hour to marinate.

2. Put the marinated chicken on a preheated grill over medium-high flame. Grill each side for 8 minutes. Allow to cool before cutting into thin slices.

3. Mix all the salad ingredients in a bowl and put the chicken on top.

4. Put all the ingredients for the dressing in a jar. Cover the jar and shake to mix thoroughly. Pour the dressing over the salad. Sprinkle with peanuts on top before serving.

Tuna Salad

Yield: 8 servings

Ingredients:

- 4 ounces green beans, cut in half

- 3 hard-boiled eggs, peeled and sliced

- 6 small new red potatoes, scrubbed and quartered

- 1 12-ounce can albacore tuna (water-packed), drained

- 2 ripe tomatoes, cored and sliced into 8 pieces

- 1/4 cup black olives, sliced

- 1/4 red onion, thinly sliced

- 1 medium head butter lettuce, rinsed, dried, and torn

For the vinaigrette:

- 2 garlic cloves, chopped

- 1 lemon, juiced

- 1 teaspoon agave nectar

- 1/4 cup red wine vinegar

- 1/2 cup olive oil

- 1/2 teaspoon sea salt

- 1 tablespoon Dijon mustard

- 1 teaspoon Herbes de Provence

Directions:

1. Boil salted water in a large pot. Cook the red potatoes for 8 minutes. Drain water. Pour a bit of olive oil over the potatoes and toss.

2. Lay the lettuce leaves on a platter. Add the eggs, tuna, red onion, tomatoes, steamed green beans, cooked potatoes, and olives.

3. Put all the ingredients for the vinaigrette in a food processor, except for the olive oil. Process until mixed. Gradually add the oil and continue mixing until everything is combined.

4. Serve the salad along with the vinaigrette.

Steak Salad with Avocado and Blue Cheese

Yield: 6 servings

Ingredients:

- 1/4 cup sliced green onions

- 4 cups mixed salad greens

- 4 ounces blue cheese, crumbled

- 1 medium avocado, diced

- 1/2 cup fresh blueberries, rinsed

- 1 pound lean steak, grilled and sliced into strips

- 1/2 cup Greek yogurt blue cheese dressing

Directions:

1. Arrange the salad greens on a platter. Add the green onion, blueberries, crumbled blue cheese, avocado, and steak slices. Pour the dressing on top of the salad. Serve immediately.

Grilled Shrimp Salad with Greek Vinaigrette

Yield: 6 servings

Ingredients:

- 3 cups whole fresh baby spinach leaves

- 2 tomatoes, thinly sliced into wedges

- 2 garlic cloves, minced

- 1 pound fresh shrimp, peeled and deveined

- 1/4 teaspoon sea salt

- 1/2 teaspoon lemon zest

- 1/3 cup Kalamata olives

- 3 cups romaine lettuce, torn

- 1/4 cup red onion, chopped

- 1 cucumber, peeled and sliced

- 1 tablespoon butter, melted

- 1/4 cup reduced-fat feta cheese

For the Greek vinaigrette:

- 1 tablespoon each of chopped fresh oregano, red wine vinegar, agave nectar, chopped fresh mint, and lemon juice

- 1/4 teaspoon freshly ground black pepper

- 1/2 teaspoon sea salt

- 3 tablespoons olive oil

Directions:

1. Wash the shrimp and pat to dry. Put them in a bowl. Add salt, butter, garlic, and lemon zest. Toss to coat. Cover the bowl and leave for 30 minutes.

2. In another bowl, mix the romaine lettuce, spinach, red onion, olives, cucumber, and tomatoes. Set aside.

3. Insert shrimp onto 4 skewers. Put them on a pre-heated grill and cook each side for 8 minutes.

4. Put all the ingredients for the vinaigrette in a food processor. Process until combined. Pour this over the salad. Top with grilled shrimp and feta cheese.

Grilled Salmon and Avocado-Strawberry Salad

Yield: 6 servings

Ingredients:

- 4 wild Atlantic salmon fillets

- 1 avocado, cubed

- 6 cups of fresh spring lettuce mix

- 1/4 red onion, thinly sliced

- 4 ounces feta cheese, crumbled

- 1-pint strawberries, sliced

- 1/4 cup sliced almonds, toasted

For the honey glaze:

- 1/4 teaspoon sea salt

- 1 tablespoon each of lemon juice and honey

- 1 teaspoon liquid smoke

- 2 tablespoons olive oil

For the honey balsamic dressing:

- 1 tablespoon honey

- 1/4 cup olive oil

- 1/4 teaspoon garlic powder

- 2 tablespoons balsamic vinegar

- Sea salt and freshly ground black pepper to taste

- 1 teaspoon Dijon mustard

Directions:

1. Combine all the ingredients for the honey glaze in a small jar. Cover and shake until well-combined.

2. Rinse the salmon fillets and pat to dry. Coat them with a bit of olive oil. Put them on a preheated grill and cook each side for 5 minutes. Transfer them to a platter and brush with the honey. Set aside.

3. Arrange the spring mix into 4 plates. Top each plate with red onion, strawberries, sliced almonds, avocado, and cheese. Add more dressing and glaze.

Napoli Salad

Yield: 6 servings

Ingredients:

- 1 tomato, diced

- 3 chicken breasts (boneless and skinless)

- 1 red bell pepper, cored and sliced

- 1/4 cup red onion, sliced

- 6 cups fresh baby spinach leaves, rinsed and stems removed

- 1/2 cup feta cheese, crumbled

- 1/3 cup bacon, cooked and crumbled

- 1 14-ounce can artichoke hearts, drained and sliced

For the balsamic vinaigrette:

- 2 garlic cloves, minced

- 1/4 cup balsamic vinegar

- 1/2 teaspoon sea salt

- 1 tablespoon Dijon mustard

- 1/2 cup olive oil

- 1/2 teaspoon dried oregano leaves

Directions:

1. Put the meat in between layers of plastic wrap. Flatten the meat by pounding using a mallet. Transfer the chicken to a bowl. Season with salt and pepper.

2. Cook each side of the seasoned chicken on a preheated grill for 5 minutes. Let stand for 5 minutes before cutting 8 slices per chicken breast.

3. Place the spinach leaves on a platter. Add tomatoes, red onion, chicken slices, crumbled bacon, artichoke hearts, feta cheese, and bell pepper.

4. Put the mustard, vinegar, salt, oregano, and garlic in a bowl. Whisk until mixed. Gradually add olive oil while whisking. Pour the vinaigrette over the salad. Toss the ingredients until combined.

Bean Salad with Grilled Flank Steak

Yield: 6 servings

Ingredients:

- 1/2 teaspoon steak seasoning

- 3 tablespoons reduced-sodium soy sauce

- Cooking spray

- 1/4 red onion, thinly sliced

- 1 pound flank steak, trimmed

- 1 15-ounce can black beans, drained and rinsed

- 1 15-ounce can white beans, drained and rinsed

- 1/2 cup roasted red bell peppers, chopped

- 1 tablespoon Worcestershire sauce

- 2 cups fresh green beans, sliced

For the balsamic dressing:

- 2 tablespoons extra virgin olive oil

- 1/4 teaspoon dried oregano

- 3 tablespoons balsamic vinegar

- 1/4 cup reduced-fat Feta cheese, crumbled

- Sea salt and freshly ground black pepper to taste

Directions:

1. Mix the Worcestershire sauce, pepper, and salt in a bowl. Generously rub all sides of the meat with the mixture. Place the seasoned meat inside a Ziploc bag, seal and refrigerate for 30 minutes.

2. Cook each side of the steak on a preheated grill for 8 minutes. Once done, transfer the meat to a chopping board and cover with loose foil. Leave for 10 minutes before cutting into thin slices.

3. Steam the green beans until crisp. Soak in a bowl filled with cold water to stop from cooking. Drain and pat dry.

4. Put the green beans in a bowl. Add the black beans, white beans, red onion, red pepper, and flank steak. Gently mix to combine.

5. In another bowl, mix the vinegar and the rest of the ingredients, except for the feta cheese. Mix well. Pour the mixture over the salad. Toss to combine. Sprinkle feta cheese on top. Cover the bowl and chill before serving.

Cobb Salad Southwestern Style

Yield: 10 servings

Ingredients:

- 1 pound chicken, cooked seasoned with taco seasoning

- 1/2 red bell pepper, seeded and diced

- 1 bag mixed salad greens

- 4 slices bacon, cooked and crumbled

- 1 15-ounce can low-sodium black beans, drained and rinsed

- 1 small avocado, diced

- 1 cup Mexican style cheese, shredded

- 1/2 cup cilantro lime ranch dressing

- 1 cup grape tomatoes, halved

For the cilantro lime ranch dressing

- 2 tomatillos, husked and quartered

- 1 cup buttermilk

- 1/4 bunch fresh cilantro

- 1 cup light mayonnaise

- 1/2 fresh lime, juiced

- 1 garlic clove

- 1 pack of Ranch Buttermilk Recipe dressing mix

- 1 jalapeno pepper, seeded and halved

Directions:

1. Put the salad greens on a platter. Put the rest of the ingredients, except for the dressing, on top.

2. Put all the ingredients for the dressing in a food processor. Process until blended. Pour this over the salad. Toss to combine.

Mediterranean Tuna Salad

Yield: 6 servings

Ingredients:

- 1/3 cup Greek olives, sliced

- 2 6-ounce cans albacore tuna, drained

- 1/2 red onion, finely sliced

- 1/2 14-ounce can artichoke hearts, drained and quartered

- 2 tablespoons flat-leaf parsley, chopped

- 1 tablespoon fresh oregano, chopped

- 2 garlic cloves, minced

- 1/4 cup red bell pepper, chopped

- Salt and freshly ground pepper to taste

- 2 tablespoons chopped fresh basil

- 2 tablespoons lemon juice

- 1/4 cup light mayonnaise

Directions:

1. Put all the ingredients in a bowl. Toss to combine.

Asian Salad with Grilled Shrimp

Yield: 6 servings

Ingredients:

- 3/4 cup Thai Peanut Dressing, divided

- 1 pound large fresh shrimp, peeled and deveined

- 2 tablespoons each of fresh lime juice, creamy peanut butter, and unseasoned rice vinegar

- 1 tablespoon each of chopped fresh mint leaves, reduced-sodium soy sauce, chopped fresh ginger, and honey

- 1 teaspoon sea salt

- 2 garlic cloves, chopped

- 1 teaspoon red pepper flakes, crushed

- 1/4 cup olive oil

For the salad:

- 1/2 cup shredded carrots

- 4 ounces baby spring mix lettuce

- 1/2 cup cucumber, thinly sliced

- 1/4 cup each of chopped fresh basil, sliced green onions, and chopped fresh cilantro leaves

- 1/2 cup sliced each yellow and red bell peppers

Directions:

1. Prepare the Thai peanut dressing. Put the following in a food processor with a metal blade attachment: soy sauce, red pepper flakes, ginger, salt, oil, vinegar, peanut butter, garlic, honey, mint leaves, and lime juice. Process until smooth.

2. Put 3/4 cup of the dressing and shrimp inside a Ziploc bag. Seal the bag and leave to marinate for 30 minutes. Put the shrimp on 4 skewers. Cook on a preheated grill for 8 minutes. Transfer to a plate and allow to cool.

3. Arrange the salad ingredients on a plate. Drizzle with the remaining dressing and top with the grilled shrimp before serving.

Seeds and Greens Salad

Yield: 6 servings

Ingredients:

- 1 teaspoon Herbes de Provence

- 2 cups butternut squash, diced

- 1 cup pomegranate seeds

- 1 tablespoon olive oil

- 1/2 cup feta cheese, crumbled

- 1/4 cup toasted pumpkin seeds

- 4 cups mixed leafy greens

For the balsamic dressing:

- 2 teaspoons Dijon mustard

- 1/2 teaspoon sea salt

- 2 garlic cloves

- 1/4 teaspoon freshly ground black pepper

- 1/2 cup olive oil

- 1/4 cup balsamic vinegar

- 1 teaspoon Herbes de Provence

- 1 tablespoon agave nectar

Directions:

1. Put the butternut squash on a baking sheet and spread all over. Sprinkle Herbes de Provence and olive oil on top. Toss to coat. Roast in a preheated oven at 425 degrees for 15 minutes. Flip them and continue roasting for 15 more minutes. Place on a wire rack to cool.

2. Put the mixed greens in a bowl. Add the pumpkin seeds, pomegranate seeds, feta cheese, and roasted squash.

3. Put all the ingredients for the dressing in a food processor. Process until smooth. Pour this over the salad. Gently mix before serving.

22 - Gastric Sleeve Diet Main Dish Recipes

Baked Pork Chops with Fruity Slaw

Yield: 4 servings

Ingredients:

- 4 center cut pork chops

- Cooking spray

- 1/2 cup low-fat evaporated canned milk

- 1/2 teaspoon garlic powder

- 1 tablespoon olive oil

- Sea salt and freshly ground black pepper to taste

- 1/2 cup Italian seasoned breadcrumbs

For the apple pear slaw:

- 1 pear, grated

- 1 apple, grated

- 2 tablespoons low-sugar apricot preserves

Directions:

1. Put the milk in a shallow dish. In another shallow dish, mix the garlic, salt, pepper, and breadcrumbs.

2. Dip the meat in the milk until all sides are covered. Dredge it in the bread crumb mixture until evenly coated. Do this with all the pieces of meat.

3. Heat oil in a pan over medium-high flame. Cook the breaded pork chop until all sides are browned. Transfer the browned pork chops on a greased baking sheet. Bake in a preheated oven at 350 degrees for 30 minutes.

4. Put the baked meat on a plate. Pour the extra juices on top. Loosely cover with foil and leave for 5 minutes to rest.

5. Combine all the ingredients for the slaw. Put a spoonful of the slaw at the top of each pork chop before serving.

Slow Cooker Pulled Pork

Yield: 10 servings

Ingredients:

- 1 cup chicken broth

- 1 onion, thinly sliced

- 2 teaspoons sea salt

- 3 garlic cloves, thinly sliced

- 1/2 teaspoon each of ground cinnamon and ground cumin

- 1 boneless pork roast

- 1 tablespoon each of chili powder and brown sugar

- 2 cups barbecue sauce

Directions:

1. Arrange the garlic and onion in a single layer at the bottom of the slow cooker. Add the broth.

2. In a bowl, mix the cinnamon, salt, cumin, chili powder, and sugar. Generously rub the pork with the mixture. Put the meat in the slow cooker. Close the lid and cook for up to 6 hours on a high setting.

3. Transfer the cooked meat to a bowl. Strain the cooking liquid from the slow cooker. Add the solid particles to the meat. Set aside the strained liquid.

4. Shred the meat and discard excess fat. Add the sauce and mix well.

This is best served with baked potato sweet fries or coleslaw.

Bacon and Beef Stew

Yield: 8 servings

Ingredients:

- 5 cups beef broth, divided

- 5 bacon slices, sliced into small pieces

- 1/2 cup flour

- 3 pounds sirloin beef, sliced into cubes

- 3 garlic cloves, minced

- 1 onion, cut into wedges

- 1 teaspoon each of thyme, oregano, and rosemary

- 2 tablespoons tomato paste

- Sea salt and freshly ground pepper to taste

- 1/2 pound carrots, rinsed and sliced diagonally

- 1 pound whole mushrooms, quartered

- 2 bay leaves

- 3 celery ribs, rinsed and sliced

- 1 pound potatoes, rinsed and cut into cubes

Directions:

1. Put the flour in a shallow dish and dredge the meat until evenly coated.

2. Put the bacon in a soup pot over medium-high heat.

Cook until crisp. Transfer to a plate lined with paper towels. Sear the coated meat in the bacon drippings until all sides are browned. Transfer to another plate.

3. Saute the garlic, onion, celery, and carrots in the same soup pot. Cook for 5 minutes before adding the beef broth. Scrape the bits at the bottom of the pot using a metal spatula. Bring to a boil. Stir in the tomato paste. Add the potato, mushrooms, bay leaves, rosemary, oregano, thyme, cooked beef and bacon, and the rest of the beef broth. Bring to a boil. Turn the heat to low and cover the pot. Simmer for 2 hours while occasionally stirring.

4. Remove the bay leaves and season with salt and pepper before serving.

Zucchini Lasagna

Yield: 8 servings

Ingredients:

- 1 6-ounce can tomato paste

- 1 15-ounce can Italian stewed tomatoes

- 2 1/2 cups zucchini, sliced lengthwise

- 1/2 cup onion, chopped

- 1/4 cup water

- 1 tablespoon each of chopped fresh oregano and chopped fresh basil leaves

- 1 pound extra-lean ground beef

- 1 egg

- 2 garlic cloves, minced

- Cooking spray

- Sea salt and freshly ground black pepper to taste

- 1/4 cup shaved Parmesan cheese

- 1 cup low-fat ricotta cheese

- 2 tablespoons chopped fresh Italian-leaf parsley

- 1 cup shredded mozzarella cheese, divided

Directions:

1. Cook the zucchinis and transfer to a plate lined with paper towels to remove excess moisture.

2. Put the meat, garlic, and onions in a pan over medium-high heat. Cook until the meat is browned on all sides. Drain the fat. Add basil, tomato paste, water, oregano, and tomatoes. Season with salt and pepper. Stir to combine and bring to a boil. Turn the heat to low and simmer for 2 minutes.

3. In a bowl, mix the beaten egg, parsley, 1/2 cup of shredded mozzarella cheese, and ricotta cheese.

4. Put 1/3 of the meat mixture on the bottom of a greased baking dish. Top with half of the zucchini slices. Add half of the ricotta cheese mixture. Add the rest of the ingredients following the same sequence. Bake in a preheated oven at 375 degrees for 30 minutes. Spread the rest of the mozzarella and parmesan cheese on top. Bake for another 10 minutes. Leave for 10 minutes before serving.

Grilled Tilapia with Papaya Salsa

Yield: 4 servings

Ingredients:

- 4 4 ounce tilapia fillets

- 1/4 cup extra-virgin olive oil

- 1 lemon, juiced

- 1 garlic clove, minced

- Sea salt and freshly ground black pepper to taste

- 2 tablespoons each of chopped fresh basil and chopped fresh Italian parsley

For the papaya salsa:

- 1 fresh lime, juiced

- 1/2 cup red onion, diced

- 1/2 cup red bell pepper, cubed

- 1/2 cup fresh cilantro, chopped

- 1 papaya, diced

- 1 jalapeno pepper, seeded and minced

Directions:

1. In a bowl, mix the lemon juice, olive oil, salt, pepper, basil, parsley, and garlic. Transfer to a Ziploc bag. Add the fish fillets. Seal the bag and marinate for an hour.

2. Put all the ingredients for the salsa, except for the papaya, in the food processor. Process until chopped. Transfer to a bowl and fold in the diced papaya.

3. Drain excess liquid from the tilapia fillets. Cook on a preheated and lightly oiled grill for 4 minutes on each side.

4. Serve the tilapia fillets with the papaya salsa on the side.

Tuna Casserole with Cheese

Yield: 6 servings

Ingredients:

- 3 6-ounce cans tuna, drained and flaked

- 1 tablespoon each of diced onion and butter

- 1/2 cup frozen petite green peas

- 2 tablespoons each of light mayonnaise and chopped celery

- 1/4 teaspoon black pepper

- 1/2 teaspoon salt

- 1 cup reduced-fat cheddar cheese, shredded

- 1/2 teaspoon garlic powder

- 1/3 cup reduced-fat cream cheese

Directions:

1. Melt butter in a pan over medium-high heat. Saute the onion and celery for 3 minutes.

2. Transfer the cooked celery and onion to a bowl. Add mayonnaise, tuna, green peas, salt, pepper, cream cheese, and garlic powder. Mix well. Transfer to a casserole dish. Top with cheese. Bake in a preheated oven at 375 degrees for 20 minutes. Leave to rest for

5 minutes before serving.

Salmon Burgers

Yield: 4

Ingredients:

- 1 pound salmon fillets, skinned and minced

- 1 egg, lightly beaten

- 1/4 cup each of red and yellow bell pepper, diced

- 1 garlic clove, minced

- 1/4 teaspoons salt

- 1/4 cup panko crumbs

- 2 teaspoons soy sauce

- Cooking spray

- 2 tablespoons chopped onion

- 1/2 teaspoons fresh lemon juice

For the lemon basil mayonnaise:

- 1 teaspoon Dijon mustard

- 2 garlic cloves, minced

- 1/2 cup light mayonnaise

- 1/2 teaspoon lemon pepper

- 1 teaspoon fresh lemon juice

- 1 teaspoon dried basil

Directions:

1. In a bowl, mix the salmon, peppers, garlic, and panko. In another bowl, mix salt, soy sauce, lemon juice, and egg. Combine the 2 mixtures. Use your hands to form 4 patties.

2. Lightly grease a skillet over medium-high heat. Cook each side of the patty for 5 minutes.

3. Combine all the ingredients for the lemon basil mayonnaise in a bowl.

4. Serve the patties along with the mayo.

Pesto Fish Roll-Ups

Yield: 4 servings

Ingredients:

- 4 4-ounce fish fillets, such as cod or flounder

- 1 tablespoon olive oil

- 1/4 cup shredded carrot

- 1/4 cup basil pesto

- Cooking spray

- 2 garlic cloves, minced

- Sea salt and freshly ground black pepper to taste

- 2 tablespoons panko breadcrumbs

- 1/4 cup finely chopped pecans

- 1/2 teaspoons lemon zest

Directions:

1. Rinse the fillets and pat them dry. Spread one side with 1 tablespoon of basil pesto. Sprinkle a tablespoon of shredded carrot on top. Roll up the fish and secure the ends with toothpicks. Arrange them in an oiled baking dish. Lightly brush with olive oil.

2. In a bowl, mix the lemon zest, panko bread crumbs, pecans, salt, pepper, and garlic. Press the mixture on top of the fish roll-ups. Bake in a preheated oven at 375 degrees for 25 minutes.

Spaghetti Squash

Yield: 6 servings

Ingredients:

- 2 tomatoes, diced

- 2 pounds spaghetti squash, halved and seeded

- 1 zucchini, diced

- Sea salt and freshly ground black pepper to taste

- 2 tablespoons olive oil, divided

- 1/2 cup shaved Parmesan cheese

- 1/2 red onion, thinly sliced

- 1/4 cup fresh basil leaves, chopped and divided

- 2 garlic cloves, minced

Directions:

1. Arrange the squash with the cut sides facing down in a baking dish. Pour 1/4 cup of water and cover. Microwave for 12 minutes on a high setting.

2. Heat a tablespoon of olive oil in a skillet over medium-high flame. Cook the garlic and onion for 3 minutes. Stir in the zucchini and cook for 3 more minutes. Add 2 tablespoons of basil leaves, tomatoes, and season with salt and pepper. Turn the heat to low and simmer for 10 minutes.

3. Scrape the strands of squash to a bowl. Add the rest of the olive oil and toss to coat. Drizzle with the vegetable mixture on top. Garnish with cheese and the

rest of the basil leaves before serving.

Caribbean Chicken

Yield: 6 servings

Ingredients:

- 1 pound chicken tenders

- 1/2 cup honey

- 1 tablespoon butter

- 1/4 cup currants

- 1/4 cup minced onion

- 1/4 cup Dijon mustard

- 1/4 cup mango chutney

- 2 garlic cloves, minced

- 1/2 teaspoon salt

- 1 teaspoon curry powder

Directions:

1. Melt butter in a pan over medium-high flame. Saute the garlic and onion for 2 minutes. Add the meat and cook until all sides are browned.

2. In a bowl, mix the mustard, honey, salt, curry, currants, and chutney. Pour this over the meat and stir. Cover the pan. Turn the heat to medium and simmer for 10 minutes.

23 - Conclusion

Thank you again for buying this book!

I hope this book was able to help you to easily cope with your life after the gastric sleeve surgery. I hope that this book also gives you ideas on what to eat and how to prepare different dishes that will fit your new dietary requirements.

Thank You

As we reach the end of this book, I want to say thanks for reading this book.

I want to get this information out to as many people as possible. If you found this book helpful, I would greatly appreciate you leaving me a review. This helps others find the book as well.

This book was self-published with the amazing help of Self-Publishing Made Easy Now! [3] . You can grab a free copy of the checklist that started my journey here: FREE Self-Publishing Checklist [4] .

[3] https://selfpublishingmadeeasynow.com/xpjv
[4] https://selfpublishingmadeeasynow.com/free_checklist

Disclaimer

This document is geared towards providing exact and reliable information in regards to the topic and issue covered. The publication is sold on the idea that the publisher is not required to render an accounting, officially permitted, or otherwise, qualified services. If advice is necessary, legal, financial, medical or professional, a practiced individual in the profession should be ordered.

This information is not presented by a financial or medical practitioner and is for entertainment, educational and informational purposes only. The content is not intended as a substitute for professional medical advice, diagnosis, or treatment. Always seek the advice of your physician or other qualified health care provider with any questions you may have regarding a medical condition. Never disregard professional medical advice or delay in seeking it because of something you have read.

The information provided herein is stated to be truthful and consistent, in that any liability, in terms of inattention or otherwise, by any usage or abuse of any policies, processes, or directions contained within is the solitary and utter responsibility of the recipient reader. Under no circumstances

www.ingramcontent.com/pod-product-compliance
Lightning Source LLC
LaVergne TN
LVHW020726200726
843506LV00009B/634